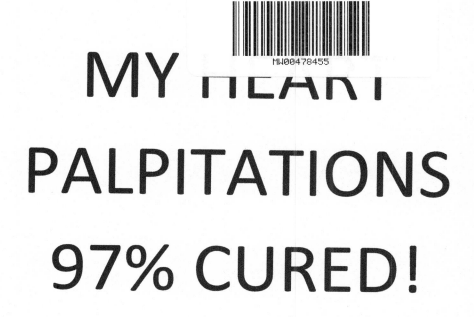

MY HEART PALPITATIONS 97% CURED!

HOW I BEAT MY HEART PALPITATIONS WITHOUT THE DOCTOR'S HELP

THE TRUE STORY OF HOW AUSTIN WINTERGREEN WENT FROM DEBILITATING HEART PALPITATIONS TO LIVING LIFE ON HIS TERMS

BY AUSTIN WINTERGREEN

Edgar Quicksand & Sons Book Publishing
Scottsdale, Arizona

Interior Layout by Sandeep Likhar
Cover Design by Gus Tikno

ISBN:

www.AustinWintergreen.com

Note from the author

Dear Reader,

Thank you for your interest in this book. I greatly appreciate it.

May I ask you a favor?

If you should come across any spelling or grammatical errors that are upsetting to you, could you please email me personally before expressing your disappointment on Amazon?

I put a lot of effort into making sure this book is free of errors, but some are bound to get through. I have personally read this book a dozen times. I've paid two professional proofreaders to catch any mistakes. I've had friends and colleagues do a read-through also.

And guess what?

I still found some mistakes when I read this book on Kindle! Ugh! As an author, this is so frustrating. As a reader, it is equally frustrating. So, if you could let me know about any spelling or grammatical errors, I'd greatly appreciate it. Here is my personal email address: austinwintergreen@gmail.com

Thank you!

Austin Wintergreen

SPECIAL DEDICATION

Thank you to all those who emailed me and let me know about various spelling errors. Your efforts are greatly appreciated!

SPECIAL APPRECIATION

Thank you to everyone who reached out to me with your stories and questions. I greatly appreciate the time you took to write me and tell me your stories. I am incredibly happy that my book is making an impact on people everywhere who suffer from heart palpitations. You are not alone.

Medical Disclaimer

None of the information in this book is backed up by science, research, or by anyone in the medical community. If you have a serious heart condition—including heart palpitations—you should seek professional medical help immediately. This book details the author's personal experiences with his opinions about heart palpitations. The author is not a healthcare provider. Not even close!

The author and publisher are providing this book and its contents on an "as is" basis and make no representations or warranties of any kind with respect to this book or its contents. The author and publisher disclaim all such representations and warranties, including, for example, warranties of merchantability and healthcare for a particular purpose. In addition, the author and publisher do not represent or warrant that the information accessible via this book is accurate, complete, or current.

The statements made about products and services have not been evaluated by the U.S. Food and Drug Administration. They are not intended to diagnose, treat, cure, or prevent any condition or disease. Please consult with your own physician or healthcare specialist regarding the suggestions and recommendations made in this book.

Except as specifically stated in this book, neither the author or publisher, nor any authors, contributors, or other representatives will be liable for damages arising out of or in connection with the use of this book. This is a comprehensive limitation of liability that applies to all damages of any kind, including (without limitation) compensatory; direct, indirect or consequential damages; loss of data, income or profit; loss of or damage to property and claims of third parties.

You understand that this book is not intended as a substitute for consultation with a licensed healthcare practitioner, such as your physician. Before you begin any healthcare program, or change your lifestyle in any way, you will consult your physician or another licensed healthcare practitioner to ensure that you are in good health and that the examples contained in this book will not harm you. This book provides content related to physical and/or mental health issues. As such, use of this book implies your acceptance of this disclaimer.

Authors Note

Some profits from this book go to two charities that are near and dear to my heart. These charities are OurPlanet.com and Aspetuck Land Trust. You will see the real significance of this choice later in the book. Aquatic life is so precious to our planet. There is plenty of evidence that it is in jeopardy. And preserving open space is also essential to our health.

If you would like to know more about how your money is being contributed to these charities, please email with any questions at: AustinWintergreen@gmail.com

UPDATE:

This book has been an incredible success. If you had read an earlier version, you would have had seen a note in this section where I mentioned that ALL profits go to charities. After donating over $1,256 to charities, I am cutting back on my donations. Some of my profits will still go to charities, but some will go into my pocket. While I love giving to charities, the profits from this book have exceeded my original goal. From here on out, 50% of the profits will go to charities.

A SPECIAL NOTE

A lot of people have written to me and told me how much this book has helped them. However, many (most) of the people who had written to me also expressed that they suffer from great anxiety.

I wrote a second book that discusses anxiety as it relates to heart palpitations. The book is called: *Conquer Your Heart Palpitations!: Discover the Unconventional Solution for Everlasting Relief.* You can find it on Amazon. It is a great complement to the book you have in your hand. If you have anxiety associated with your heart palpitations, I strongly suggest you take a look at it.

Table of Contents

Preface

I've wanted to write this book for a very long time. The reason being is that if I could write a book such as this one, that would mean that I was cured of my heart palpitations. That was the promise I made to myself. No cure? No book. No blabbing.

I had found a great many things to help me on my journey of being cured. I vowed that I couldn't talk about any of these remedies until I cured myself.

Please note that this book is about my personal journey toward a full cessation of heart palpitations. Therefore, I have not done any additional research other than what I had already done. Everything you read is from my head. Consequently, you won't find any references to science to back up what I am claiming in this book.

Let's be clear. Everything I tell you about here happened to me. Many people write books about heart palpitations and list a bunch of solutions. However, they never experienced them. They just got stuff off the Internet and regurgitated them. I didn't. Every symptom mentioned I have experienced. Every vitamin listed I tried. Every mind-body solution I have practiced. This is my story. Not someone else's or embellished in any way.

Short book

I tried hard to keep this book as quick as possible. I know many authors want to make their books long to make them seem more credible. Well, I'm not a doctor, so legitimacy has already gone out of the window.

When I want a solution to a problem, I don't want to read a long book. I don't read a non-fiction book for the sake of reading. I read a book like this one to find a solution to my problem. Therefore, I tried to make this book as concise as possible. I didn't put in a lot of scientific studies because I would only be repeating what others have said and slowed things down. Like I mentioned before, this book is solely about my experience.

Technical terms

I don't use a lot of technical terms like heart arrhythmia, tachycardia, bradycardia, AFib, etc. They all seem the same to me. Also, I feel like I had experienced all of those. I've had irregular heartbeats. I've had slow heartbeats (bradycardia); I've had rapid heartbeats (tachycardia), and everything in between. I'm confident my remedies will work for everything and everyone.

As I said, I want to make this book as short as possible, so I don't want to get bogged down with scientific terms. I never really cared what condition a doctor said I had. I just cared about getting a solution as quickly as possible. And I believe you do too.

In fact, once you get labeled with an ailment (i.e., tachycardia), it will make it harder for you to recover. You will use that term, tachycardia, to identify yourself. Research has shown that people who are labeled and identify with a particular ailment recover more slowly. It has to do with the nocebo effect, which is the opposite of the placebo effect.

You have a heartbeat issue. Let's leave it at that and find a solution. How does that sound? Sounds good to me, too!

SECTION I

Introduction

I'm sure you are frustrated with your condition.

I know I was. I couldn't do anything. I had to give up so many things that I love. I used to play tennis every week. I had to give that up because my heart couldn't take any exercise. I used to work out every day at the gym. Couldn't do that anymore.

I loved swimming in the ocean. Couldn't do that anymore. In fact, one of my most significant heart palpitation episodes took place while I was frolicking in the ocean. Yes, I was frolicking. I wasn't really swimming. I was just goofing off, but then suddenly, my heart went crazy, beating at 170 beats a minute.

You probably had to give up things that you love as well.

My condition was so bad that I couldn't even roll over in my bed without my heart going crazy. I'm sure you've had similar experiences. I've heard about them on Facebook and YouTube.

My Biggest Frustration

My biggest frustration with heart palpitations support groups on Facebook is that no one listened to my advice. I've been commenting on Facebook and YouTube and on forums about heart palpitations. But no one wants to listen to me. They just want sympathy. That's what it comes down to. However, I will tell you this now and later in the book, seeking sympathy is the LAST thing you want to do. It will only hamper your progress.

I ask you to read this book with an open mind. Many things that I write about here are my personal experiences, so you may not have heard of these solutions. It will automatically make you say, "I never heard that before. That's doesn't sound right." You must trust me. I had horrible and debilitating heart palpitations. Now I'm 97% cured.

I read some whacky things in other books. Guess what? I tried many of them. Some of them worked!

I congratulate you on continuing your search to find a solution to your problem. It shows that you are committed to solving your problem. In my experience, you need to have a constant commitment to resolving your issue if you want to get better. Many well-meaning people told me, "It's harmless. There's no cure. It's something you just will have to live with."

Do you know what my response was? "Forget that! I wasn't born with this, and it didn't come from outer space. I did something to cause this. I'm gonna do something to un-cause this!"

Why 97% cured?

Although on most days I feel fantastic like my old self, they are sometimes (very rarely) where I get a little reminder of my condition. It's not a heart palpitation, but it's just a small bump. It's kind of like a quarter skip.

Here's a comparison. In music, you have whole notes, half notes, and quarter notes. The beats that I feel in my chest are like quarter notes. I wouldn't notice it at all if I never had this condition. That's why I call it a reminder.

I can do nearly everything I did before the onslaught of my heart palpitations.

Please note that since my cure, I haven't gone back to my old ways. I still eat healthy meals, take vitamins and supplements. Most of this is not only necessary for my heart palpitations but also for my overall health. You would think that if you were cured, you could go back to their old way of living.

The answer to that is yes and no. If you were cured of malaria, I wouldn't recommend going back to hanging around mosquitoes. If you got triple bypass surgery, I wouldn't recommend that you open a fried chicken and waffle stand. If you got gastric bypass surgery, I wouldn't recommend that you make plans to attack a dozen all-you-can-eat buffets in the next month.

Although I still take supplements, maintain a healthy diet, and practice mind-body exercises, I still consider myself cured. I don't find myself "maintaining" my condition like someone who is maintaining their high blood pressure or cholesterol. Those meds are only for those conditions. The remedies in this book serve more than just a floppy heart. (See? I'm not using technical terms.)

Usually, these reminders happen when I go out on a bender. What is a bender? Well, it's either drinking a bunch of beers and vodka tonics with my buddies or hitting the Dunkin' Donuts for some coffee loaded with sugar and cream—with one or two donuts on the side. I gotta live. I'm no saint, but I am saintly.

Why this book is different

Most books I've read about heart palpitations come from doctors, nutritionists, or well-meaning opportunists. That's okay. They have some excellent information in them—especially if you haven't read anything else on this topic before.

However, they all repeat the same information. Why? Because they are all getting that information from the same source— namely the Internet. This book is all about *my* experience. I didn't put anything in this book that I didn't experience myself—even if I thought it was helpful.

In other words, I've come across a lot of tips on the Internet about resolving heart palpitations. Unless I've personally tried it, I won't make you read about it in this book. You've probably have heard it before.

I can guarantee that you haven't heard a lot about what you are going to read in this book.

-1-

My Story from the Beginning Until Now

I think my account will help you identify with the many frustrations you currently have. I know it helped me to read, listen, and watch other people's stories about their heart palpitations.

Reading other people's stories was more important than reading an article or watching a video from a doctor. Even the doctors who addressed my issue with heart palpitations didn't seem to be sympathetic. I was dying here! At least that's what I thought every time my heart bounced around like a wild animal in my chest.

Hearing other people's stories made me feel like I wasn't alone with my condition, which my regular doctors seemed to ignore. It still amazes me that so many people have this problem, but regular physicians seem to be so clueless about it. Crazy, isn't it?

The viral infection that started it all

My heart palpitations started in earnest four years ago (2016) after I was recovering from a viral infection. My viral infection was so bad that I had to go to the emergency room. My eyes were bleeding. I had welts all over my body. I had trouble breathing. My wrist and ankles ached so severely that I had to walk up the stairs on my elbows and knees. My head felt like it was going to explode from all the pressure on my brain.

My viral infection was so obscure that they just called it a "viral infection." They didn't give it a name like Tuberculosis, pneumonia, measles, polio, rabies, Ebola, backwater Flu, or anything else. Months after my release from the hospital, I did some research on my condition with all the symptoms I had. The closest thing I could come up with was rheumatic fever. That's just me playing doctor. Anyway, I had a nasty viral infection.

They treated me with all sorts of drugs in which I took intravenously. One drug felt like morphine or something. For a brief moment, I was in a total state of bliss. Nothing else mattered. However, it was only for a brief moment. Then I was back to the swollen head and achy joints.

The beginning of the heart palpitations

It wasn't until after I came out of the hospital that my heart palpitations were out of control. For months, I blamed my viral infection for the cause of my heart palpitations. Then later, I blamed all the antibiotics they gave me.

To this day, I don't have substantial evidence either way. Still, I tend to think it was the antibiotics that may have exacerbated my heart palpitations because my stomach flora has never been the same. I have a fair amount of bathroom issues even though I eat fiber like it's going out of stock. Anyway, we will read later about how I finally got over that!

My focus was not so much to find the cause of my heart palpitations; it was to find a solution. In retrospect, maybe if I had spent a little more time on the cause, I may have found a solution sooner. I don't know. You never know about these things. Anyway, I was extremely impatient, so I set out to find a solution.

The unlikely solution

The first "solution" came in the form of magnesium. I read several articles and watched several videos about this miracle mineral. Remember, it's a mineral, not a vitamin.

So, what did I do when I learned of this miracle mineral? I went out got me some magnesium. Yes'm. That's what I did. I went down to my local CVS and bought me some magnesium. I took a tablet or two and then waited.

Guess what?

It worked! It really worked!

My heart palpitations subsided.

What a miracle. End of book, right? What else could be on the rest of these pages?

Well, as I will mention over and over again in this book, many of the remedies I took had a placebo effect. They would work for two weeks, and then my heart palpitations came back.

So, the magnesium wasn't quite the miracle I was hoping it would be. Later in the book, I will discuss in more detail my magnesium regiment and why I still take magnesium. For now, let's move on with my heart palpitations escapades!

Unforeseen triggers

During my research, I learned about the triggers for my heart palpitations. You may have heard about many of these. The most common are caffeine, alcohol, and sugar. They deplete magnesium and other vitamins and minerals. I will go into a lot more detail about triggers later in this book. I will discuss many you may not have heard—especially one that is very common in salad dressings and potato chips!

At this point, I gave up coffee, ice cream, and... that's it. That was about as far as I got. I still drank alcohol—even hard liquor. Today, I don't drink that much.

When I quit caffeine and reduced my sugar load, I felt better. My heart palpitations went away... for about two weeks. Later they came back.

In another chapter, I will explain how I gave up coffee and how I learned to love herbal tea.

Quitting coffee was still good for me even though my heart palpitations subsided only a little. However, at this point, I was getting very frustrated with my progress. I thought I was doing everything I needed to do. I got rid of the triggers. I was taking magnesium just like everyone had suggested. What else was there to do?

Every time I had a heart palpitation, I would curse the world. I was pissed. I would yell, "Fuck this shit!" over and over. Fortunately, I was self-employed and working out of my home, so I was allowed to yell out profanities at will.

However, I will later learn that this was very detrimental to finding my cure. I will discuss later in this book how having the proper mindset will make all the difference in your progress in finding your cure.

At this point, I was looking for new ways to help with my cure. So far, I was taking supplements (more than just magnesium). I had nearly completely quit coffee and caffeine. I had significantly reduced my sugar and alcohol intake. I was about 54% cured at this point. I was happy but still frustrated. I had made lots of progress but still needed more to go.

Revolutionary diet (not really)

I did stumble upon one dietary remedy that skyrocketed my progress. I found this remedy entirely by accident.

One night I was having dinner with my wife. I ate a dish that had a lot of onions in it. I drank a considerable about of beer that evening, and I feared that I would have many heart episodes the following morning. Guess what? I didn't.

I attributed my lack of heart palpitations to the onions.

A few days went by, and my heart palpitations came back with a vengeance. This was when I devised a sweet dish that would bring me to about 69% cured.

Usually, I would have two eggs and red bell pepper for breakfast. But on this particular morning, I made a new dish. It consisted of sautéed broccoli, mushrooms, and onions.

After I ate this breakfast, I felt fantastic! I finally found something that gave me a tremendous amount of relief. To this day, I try to eat one whole onion every week. I have several dishes that I make with onions. Later in the book, I will go into more detail about my diet.

As usual, my new breakfast was not the panacea that I thought it was going to be. However, I did bring my palpitations down a bit and was about 73% cured.

Unfortunately, at this point, I was slacking off on the other parts of my treatment plan. With my new diet and quitting all the triggers, magnesium seemed to be a distant memory.

You see, I have the incurable habit of not making good habits. I don't seem to put everything together. I only have enough willpower to do one thing. Science says that we do have a limited capacity of willpower, and then we use it all up.

I was trying to have a supplement regime, quit a bunch of foods that I craved (and was addicted to), and trying new meals to prepare. It was all too much for me. I depleted my willpower.

Something always had to give. But I persevered.

CoQ10 and what it did to me

Once the diet was going nicely, I wanted to explore more supplements to see if any were more effective than magnesium. I found a few. During my research, I found that CoQ10 was beneficial for the heart.

When I started taking CoQ10, I found that it did indeed help with my heart palpitations. I took CoQ10 in addition to magnesium. This regime seemed to have brought my cure to about 83%. At this time, I was having very few palpitations. When I usually had hundreds a day, I was now down to dozens a day. I was improving.

However, this had also been around the one and half year mark for when my heart palpitations began in earnest. So maybe the lapse of time had something to do with it.

What I do know is that my tolerance for my heart palpitations had gone down. I couldn't take it anymore. It's kind of like a barking dog in the neighborhood or a crying baby on an airplane. At first, you can deal with it. However, the more you are exposed to it, the less you can deal with it.

My palpitations may have lessened, but they bothered me more than ever because I had tried so many remedies and felt I was so close to finding a real cure.

I wanted to find a real cure badly. I didn't want to mask my symptoms with magnesium and other supplements. I wanted an actual cure.

Anyway, by taking CoQ10 and magnesium, my palpitations reduced considerably, but they were still bothersome. They were so bothersome—and I felt I was so close to a cure—that I started overdosing on magnesium and CoQ10. I was taking twice the recommended amount of magnesium (I managed to build up a tolerance of the bathroom activities) and three times the recommended amount of CoQ10.

I wanted to put my heart issues to bed. As I will discuss later in the book, magnesium is the mineral that relaxes your muscles (i.e., your heart), whereas calcium contracts your muscles. Sometimes, I didn't even know if I had a heartbeat. Some days, I would freak out a bit, thinking my heart stopped because it was beating so softly and slowly.

Drilling a hole into my heart

Then one day, I felt a strange pain in the middle of my chest. It was as if someone was slowly drilling a hole in my heart. It wasn't excruciating; it was a mild pain. Since it was in my heart, I got a little worried.

After the third day of this, I thought maybe I had some kind of slow heart attack. I had heard of people having abdominal pain and finding out that they had a heart attack.

Thinking about this, I went to a walk-in clinic that was highly rated. The doctor asked me a bunch of questions and concluded with, "I think you might be having a heart attack. Go to the emergency room. We will call ahead. They will be expecting you."

"Good grief," I thought.

Fun times at the emergency room

I went to the emergency room. I checked in at the desk, and the woman said, "Someone will be with you shortly." I sat down, thinking I was having a heart attack. Then it dawned on me: "Why am I waiting? This is an emergency! I'm having a heart attack. Didn't they get the memo?"

I got up from my chair and said to the woman at the desk, "Didn't you get the memo? My doctor sent me here for heart trouble." I said heart trouble because I didn't want to mention heart attack out loud, thinking that maybe it would get worse if I spoke the devil's name out loud. I'm superstitious like that. The devil. (Shit, now I am bringing the devil into this. What is wrong with me?)

This is how far this whole heart trouble has taken me. I had a strange viral infection cured with antibiotics. Now, I'm in an emergency room thinking I'm having a heart attack. However, I dare not say it aloud because I might conjure up the beast of the underworld. Ugh!

Anyway, I pushed. The receptionist expedited my order (or whatever it's called). After getting my blood pressure checked by a nurse, they plopped me down in a bed in the emergency department. Good. That's where I needed to be.

The doctor came in and asked me a bunch of questions. They took my pulse and hooked me up to a blood pressure monitor that continuously took my blood pressure.

At first, my blood pressure was high. It started to come down. They took an x-ray of my chest and then made me watch daytime television. I asked for a gun so that I could shoot myself. Not because of my heart but because daytime TV is so mind-numbingly nauseating. How do people watch that crap and still live another day? I don't get it.

Anyway, everything was looking good. My chest x-ray looked good. Even the nurse put on the report that my lungs were "grossly clear." Grossly clear? What the hell does that mean?

My attending physician was at a loss for words. He didn't find anything wrong with me. I told him about my heart palpitations. He looked at me as if I said, "I have a pebble in my shoe." He couldn't figure out why I was telling him this. It was almost as if he didn't even know what "heart palpitations" were. He just looked at me blankly and left the room.

Upon my discharge, the doctor returned and said, "Well, the lab reports look good. We can't see anything wrong with you. Perhaps you had a little acid reflux."

When he said that, I just rolled my eyes. I don't eat the kind of crappy food that gives people acid reflux or "heartburn," as people like to call it. I also knew what heartburn was and what it felt like. I had it once in college. I ate a sausage po-boy, and my heart hurt like crazy. I was very familiar with heartburn.

Anyway, he gave me a Prilosec as if he didn't know what else to give me. He felt obligated to provide me with something. I just wanted to say to him, "Look, man, if there is nothing wrong with me, then don't give me anything. I'm okay with leaving with nothing. I do it all the time. I shop for clothes and leave with nothing. I'm okay with nothing. But don't give me some bullshit pill to appease me. I don't need that."

I took the pill and debated about throwing it over my shoulder right there in the emergency room. I was so insulted. However, I didn't do it because I sympathized with the doctor a little bit. Every day, whiny patients who see a doctor expect to get some medicine or a prescription. They cry if they don't at least get something.

This is what has happened to our "death care" in this country. Sometimes doing nothing is the exact medicine we need. I will talk later about how your attitude and psychology have a lot to do with your heart palpitations.

Emergency room goodbye and good riddance

I left the emergency room happy. I didn't have a heart attack, but I was pissed that the attending physician was clueless about my heart palpitations. He was an emergency room doctor, for crying out loud! He must have known something about heart palpitations, right?

When I got home, I realized I had been overdosing too much on magnesium and CoQ10, so I immediately stopped taking them. I realized I was taking three times the recommended daily amount of CoQ10 and twice the recommended daily amount of magnesium. No surprise that I was feeling a little off.

Guess what?

I felt better. I was getting closer to my cure. Wee!

But as always, after two weeks, the euphoria of being cured faded and nearly disappeared as I was having more heart palpitations.

I couldn't sleep. I couldn't exercise. I still had trouble walking upstairs and up hills without feeling breathless. I had come a long way. However, I was still troubled by my heart palpitations.

I started retaking magnesium, but I put the CoQ10 aside.

For about six months, I continued this regimen. I was taking magnesium and having an onion every week. Gave up eggs completely.

This kept my heart palpitations at bay when I wasn't doing anything. However, when I exercised, problems started up again.

The attack at the gym

I had one particularly memorable attack when I was at the gym. At the time, I was feeling good that my heart palpitations were minimal, so I started working out hard.

I ran on the treadmill, and then I started lifting weights. I made sure my breathing wasn't too heavy, as that was usually when my heart palps would begin to kick in, especially climbing more than one flight of stairs.

When I finished doing my heaving exercises, I went over to the stretching area to do some after-work-out stretches.

This was when my big attack happened.

I was sitting down quietly, stretching my legs. I leaned over, and then wham! My heart went into hyperdrive. It was pounding at about 200 beats a minute. I held my chest and just sat there thinking, "Well, this is it. This is the big one. I'm gonna die right here in this gym. Plenty of people die in gymnasiums from heart failure all the time. Why couldn't it be me?"

My heart just pounded and pounded. I was thinking about alerting someone, but I've had episodes like this before, and then everything calmed down. I just sat for a while, hoping my heart would regain a normal rhythm.

But it didn't. It just kept pounding hard and fast like a jackhammer splitting concrete.

While this was happening, I was also thinking, "My heart can't take this anymore. How can it beat so fast and not burn out?" I was comparing it to using an American hairdryer in Europe. You would blow it out because there is too much voltage. I just kept thinking that my heart wasn't designed to beat this fast. I was expecting smoke to come out of my ears like on an episode of a *Tom & Jerry* cartoon.

A woman was sitting next to me, stretching her legs. I was just about to tap her on the leg and say, "Can you call someone? I think I'm having a heart attack." I didn't want to say my heart was beating fast because she probably would have said, "No shit. You're in a gym. Join the crowd." So, I was going to cut to the chase and declare a heart attack. And there was a small part of me that was thinking heart attack.

But right at the moment of this decision to tap her on the leg, my heart calmed down and regained its normal rhythm.

What a relief!

I was so thankful that my heart had regained its normal rhythm. I just sat there in amazement as to what had happened. I was saddened because I thought I had come so far with my cure.

It seemed as if there was nothing I could do to help with my problem. I felt like I would have to deal with these heart palpitations for the rest of my life. I wouldn't be able to exercise or do anything to elevate my heart rate without going into some kind of tachycardia episode.

I was depressed after that incident.

I avoided the gym like the plague for the next three weeks. Instead of the gym, I just took light, gingerly walks on the beach. This wasn't much help. I was freaking out all the time. I felt like my heart would go into tachycardia any minute. But I wanted some exercise. I missed it.

The walks on the beach helped a little. During this time, I doubled down on my diet and supplements. Things started to improve slightly.

Learning to breathe

After that summer, I read a book about heart palpitations. In this book, the author mentioned Ayurvedic breathing. I didn't know what that was, so I looked on Amazon to see if there were any books about it.

(By the way, I use Amazon to look up info just as much as Google because I find books to be much more authoritative.

There are too many clowns posting blogs about stuff in which they know nothing. At least an author of a book has put in a little more effort into it.)

Anyway, I came upon a book called *The Oxygen Advantage* by Patrick McKeown. The book is about breathing techniques that were pioneered by Konstantin Buteyko, a Russian doctor. The method is basically to breathe less.

In Buteyko's opinion, bad health is attributed to breathing too much. And breathing through the mouth is unhealthy and causes many health problems. We are meant to breathe through our noses.

The book is really for people who have asthmas, but I read it anyway because some reviewers said it helped with their heart palpitations.

I won't explain any more than that. But I will tell you about one of the techniques that significantly improved my heart palpitations.

Patrick McKeown said to tape your mouth shut while sleeping. This sounded like a novel idea. I read this in the evening hours, so all I had was some old duct tape lying around. I taped my mouth shut for the evening.

The next day, I felt different. I didn't have that anxiety kind of feeling in my chest. My heart palpitations significantly improved. Who knew?

That day, I bought some medical tape. I planned on doing this every evening. I have been doing this nearly every evening for the past six months. It has been one of the best things I did for my journey to rid myself of heart palpitations.

At this point, I felt as if I was about 75% cured. I was feeling good. I used some other techniques that I will review later in this book.

Meditation and what it does

I had never meditated in my entire life. But when it came time to cure my ailing heart, I was willing to try anything. I don't mean to make meditation sound like some weird drastic measure. I only mean to say that it was so foreign to me.

For me, people who meditated sit on a mountaintop with their limbs crossed, eyes closed and focused on their breath. That was not me at all. I was so far from that world. My world was standing at sea level, limbs parallel, and erratic breathing. That was my world.

But I tried it. It helped a little. The whole mental thing helped a lot, but the initial mediations helped only a little. I will get into the whole psychological thing later in the book.

The strategies I used

I will continue my story further in the book as I talk about the different strategies that I used to get my heart palpitations to be 97% cured. Every one of these things did help in some small way. Some things I probably wouldn't do if I had to go through with this all over again.

Summary

I tried to give you a small glimpse of what I was going through. I didn't want to drag it out too long. But so that you know, these episodes frequently happened for three years. I couldn't roll over on my bed without my heart going into some erratic rhythm.

I will expand upon my story as I go through the different treatments that I used to get me 97% cured of my heart palpitations. Read on to get your cure!

Key takeaways:

- I suffered a lot
- I went to the emergency room
- I couldn't exercise without issues
- Magnesium helped

SECTION II
What I've Tried and What Works

-2-

Triggers

Many things can trigger your heart palpitations. I will talk about the ones that set me off regularly. Maybe you can relate. Some of these you may already know about, but some you may not. It helps to review the ones you already have and learn about the ones you don't.

Caffeine

During my research, I discovered how caffeine affects my heart palpitations. Today it seems so obvious, but before I knew what was going on, it didn't.

Caffeine is a stimulant. At that time, it was news to me because caffeine never affected me (my heart palpitations) until after I had my illness with the viral infection. Regularly, I would drink one to two cups (Starbucks medium) a day with no ill effects.

However, I found out about the severe adverse effects the hard way. One day I was driving to work drinking my coffee, and then BOOM, my heart started going into overdrive. All I could think of at the time was, "Oh boy; this is the big one."

Although I felt that I had a lot of life left in me, I had heard of many people knocking off at 46, so this sudden attack—as I like to call them—really got me scared. I want to call these episodes an attack, but unfortunately, a "heart attack" already means something else entirely.

When my heart goes a million miles a minute, it feels like an attack—more than just an episode. However, when I talk to my wife or the public, I just call it an episode. But the word episode seems so weak. It feels like an attack, doesn't it?

I pulled over to the side of the road and tried to keep myself from dying—because that's what I thought was happening. This wouldn't be the first time I thought I was dying. Nearly four years later, when I thought I had this thing licked and I considered myself close to 80% cured and knew how to handle these things, I had another episode in which I told my wife to call an ambulance. Later I realized this was all psychosomatic. She managed to talk me out of it. Wonderful wife, indeed.

Anyway, caffeine was a big culprit, which was good and bad. The bad part was I loved coffee (especially with liberal portions of cream and sugar. After all, in that form, it's really just melted coffee ice cream, which I also love because of the sugar and cream).

The good news was that as soon as I licked the coffee habit, my heart palpitations would be gone. At this point (which was about 6 months after my viral infection and taking antibiotics), my heart palpitations were not so frequent. I would play a little game of "Chicken" with myself and drink coffee even though I was running the risk of having a massive heart episode.

I tried very hard to quit coffee. I even went to a hypnotist to get over my coffee addiction. It worked, and it didn't work. It worked in that I ultimately gave up coffee, but it took nearly a year—not what the hypnotist promised. Therefore, I don't know what to say about all that. I guess she was right…eventually.

Well, the good news about caffeine and coffee having a massive effect on my heart palpitations was that all I needed to do was kick the habit. Right? Once kicked, happy days are here again. I tried hard to kick the habit.

One of the things that the hypnotist said to me was that I liked to have warm liquid flowing down my throat. This was part of the therapy sessions. Weeks later, I realized she was right. Therefore, I started drinking tea to substitute for my coffee habit. It wasn't nearly as fun, but I did it anyway.

In case you're wondering, I only drank decaffeinated and herbal teas. I didn't drink green or black tea. Anyway, this helped. I no longer had any of the heart episodes that were caused by drinking coffee.

Unfortunately, this only lasted two weeks. Then my heart palpitation came back. So far, I have tried magnesium and quitting coffee. I was really at my wit's end.

Since coffee was out, I switched to drinking hot tea. I will go more into more detail about my tea-drinking regime in another chapter. However, I will touch upon another trigger (for me, at least) that doesn't get mentioned anywhere, and that is hot foods and beverages.

Hot foods and beverages

When I switched to drinking tea, I felt a lot better. I eliminated coffee from my diet. Tea, for the most part, was going great. However, sometimes, when I drank my tea too hot, I noticed that it set off a heart palpitation.

This also held true for hot foods. If I had anything hot, like hot oatmeal, my heart would startup. I believe this had to do with the vagus nerve. I will talk about this later.

MSG

I recently read an article claiming that MSG was NOT that bad for human consumption. It sounds like someone from the MSG consortium wrote that article. In other words, I say, "Bullshit!"

MSG was indeed a trigger for me. Once I eliminated it from my diet, I felt much better. Most people think MSG is only found in Chinese food. You'd be surprised how many foods contain MSG.

I won't mention them here, but I was surprised to find that my Hidden Valley Ranch Dressing contained MSG. No wonder it was so delicious. Anyway, that went right into the trash.

It's hard to avoid MSG and other additives that affect you like MSG. The best thing to do is to do some research to find out what those foods are. I don't eat a lot of packaged foods, so I didn't dive deep into the research department. However, when I do buy something in a bottle, a jar, a can, or a box, I check the ingredients. If anything sounds funny, I look it up.

Snacks like flavored potato chips and tortilla chips often have MSG or similar flavor enhancers. Anything that sounds unnatural or exotic, like *Blaze* or *Jacked,* is most likely to have some kind of MSG in it. I'm talking to you, Doritos!

Sugar

Sugar is a big one for me. To put it simply, I love sugar. I love sugar so much it's killing me to have to give it up. I didn't really give it up, but I did reduce my intake by at least 94.3%.

I used to eat a container of Pepperidge Farm Mint Milano cookies in one sitting. I used to eat an ice cream cone every day. I used to drink coffee with enough sugar to overpower the bitterness of coffee. I used to eat boxes of Cocoa Krispies, Froot Loops, and Apple Jacks in one sitting. I used to eat a pint of mint chocolate chip gelato in one sitting. I often got a sugar hangover but never a raging heart spasm.

Now. Now, it's all over. No more cookies. No more coffee. No more cereal. No more ice cream. No more of anything that contains a nice serving of sugar.

Instead of eating sugary cereals, I have a bowl of hot oatmeal with raspberries and blueberries on top. Delicious. To sweeten my oatmeal, I mash up a near-rotten banana and mix it in while the oatmeal is cooking. It really sweetens up the grain without the need for artificial sugar.

I'm not going to lie to you; I still have sugar on occasions. However, I've made some wise choices. I told you about the banana instead of sugar. If I get a powerful craving for sugar— like I want a Snickers bar, I will get a Kind bar. Less sugar, more nuts.

I've also discovered that Kombucha is quite sweet but doesn't have a lot of sugar. I mix it with seltzer water for a nice, sweet drink. The ratio I use is one part Kombucha and five parts seltzer water.

One thing to know about sugar is that you taste it more when it is on top of your food than when you mix it in. For instance, if you are eating oatmeal and want to sweeten it with brown sugar, don't mix it in. Leave it on top.

I also noticed this phenomenon when I would put sugar in my coffee. The more I stirred my coffee after I put in my sugar, the less I tasted it. What I would do then is just stir it once or twice and then leave it alone. But as mentioned before, I no longer drink coffee.

Anyway, sugar is a big culprit because it causes the depletion of magnesium. Low magnesium is attributed to heart palpitations.

We'll talk more about this in the *Vitamins and Minerals* section of this book.

I noticed a big difference once I eliminated sugar from my diet. I have an occasional treat, but for the most part, sugar is out of my life. I was able to satisfy cravings with fruit. Fruit is much more delicious once you don't have sugar in your life.

This is probably a good time to tell you to stay away from soda in any form. It is loaded with sugar. And don't think diet sodas are any better. As we will discuss, the artificial sweeteners in diet sodas and other drinks will wreak havoc on your body.

If you do quit drinking soda, don't substitute it with fruit juices. Fruit juices are loaded with sugar. They have more sugar than soda. Don't drink this stuff, and don't give it to your kids. It is deadly.

Alcohol

They call it "holiday heart" when you have heart palpitations when you drink. The funny thing is I never got "holiday heart" while I was drinking. However, I did have it often the next day. I like my martinis every now and then. But my condition got so bad that I had to give up alcohol altogether.

As you will read later in this book, I was able to drink alcohol again when I got my condition to be about 97% cured. Actually, I never went back to the hard stuff. Now, I just drink light beers. The beers I drink the most are Coors Light and Michelob Ultra. They don't seem to give me much trouble.

One thing you need to think about when consuming alcohol is that it depletes your magnesium levels. This is why when I drink alcohol, I take an extra dose of magnesium. I usually take it with L-Theanine before I go to bed. This allows me to get a good night's sleep. I will talk more about magnesium and L-Theanine in the *Vitamins and Minerals* section of this book.

I've come a long way when it comes to alcohol. I used to drink Mojitos and Margaritas. These are loaded with sugar—and, of course, alcohol. I don't drink them much anymore these days. I just stick to my beer. I usually only have about four beers a week.

The worst kind of alcohol is liqueurs. I used to love—and still do—drinks such as Disaronno, Sambuca, Frangelico, Fireball, and Kalua. Those were the worst for me. They are nothing but sugar bombs mixed with alcohol.

If you have heart palpitations, you might want to reduce your alcohol intake because it's a major trigger for most people.

Artificial sweeteners

I used to use Equal in my coffee. My wife reminded me of the dangers of Equal and Splenda. There are several books on this topic. Once I switched from artificial sweeteners to sugar, I actually felt better. This was long before my heart palpitations started. I just felt better in my head. My mind was clearer.

Whatever you do, stay away from artificial sweeteners. They are deadly. Neurosurgeon Dr. Russell Blaylock wrote a book (actually several) on this topic. The best one I know is titled, *Excitotoxins: The Taste That Kills.* It will tell you all the facts you need to know about artificial sweeteners and how they will mess you up. You are better off with just plain white sugar.

When it comes to heart palpitations, artificial sweeteners are a significant trigger for some people. Your best bet is just to get used to enjoying sweet fruit and get over your sweet tooth. No kidding.

As discussed earlier in the sugar section, you may be drinking diet sodas and think you are doing yourself a favor. You are not. Diet sodas are horrible for you. There are several scientific studies that say diet soda actually makes you fatter.

In a nutshell, the science says that when you consume a diet soda, your body thinks it is consuming a food source. When you get no calories from that soda, your body goes looking for those calories. That leads to overeating—especially unhealthy foods.

Have you seen any thin person drink diet soda? Neither have I. In fact, skinny people don't drink soda. They know it makes you fat. This is why you will always see thin people drinking water.

One more thing about artificial sweeteners. They are finding their way into everything. Be sure to read the labels on your food. Or just do a taste test. When I eat something that tastes kind of sweet—like store-bought coleslaw, I check the label. I've had chicken salad taste sweet. Later I found out they put sugar in it. People put sugar in coleslaw. I'm not sure, but they do.

Dehydration

When it comes to heart palpitations, drink lots of fluids. You want to stay hydrated throughout the day. I know when I'm lacking water in my body, that's when I get heart palpitations. When I wake in the morning, the first thing I do is have two sixteen-ounce glasses of water. I just gulp them down. Presto!

If I don't drink a lot of water in the morning, I get dehydrated by the afternoon. I don't like to drink a lot of water in the evening because then I will have to wake up in the middle of the night to go to the bathroom.

This is another reason why I like to drink tea. Water can be bland and not fun to drink. However, tea adds a little flavor. My favorite way to drink tea and to ensure I am drinking a lot is through my ten-ounce Thermos container. I throw in one or two tea bags and then drink it throughout the day. This is very convenient when I'm in my car or at the office. I have at least three of these during the day.

At this point, I've had at least 5 sixteen-ounce glasses of water or tea. This is better than what most people drink.

I also eat a lot of fruit. My breakfast is usually made up of oatmeal and fruit. For every ½ cup of oatmeal, there is one cup of water. This is part of the reason why I like to eat oatmeal. Sometimes I have oat bran, which has a higher water ratio.

I generally don't have to worry about dehydration if I have my tea, oatmeal, and fruit.

If you are someone who eats dry foods like bagels with cream cheese, or ham and eggs, or breakfast sandwiches, you need to be taking in a lot of water to stay well hydrated. Don't think orange juice will do the trick. As said before, orange juice is loaded with sugar.

Keeping track

The right way of making sure you are getting enough water is actually to keep track. On a pad of paper, I draw eight circles. Every time I drink a glass of water, I put an X through it. This helps me keep track of the water.

There is also an app that will help you keep track, but I like to keep things simple and low-tech. However, one of these days, I might get around to downloading that app...

...okay, I just downloaded a water tracker app. I will see how it goes. There are three in the Apple store. Just look up "water tracker," and you find what you need. I can't recommend any because I haven't tried any.

Staying hydrated

One right way to stay hydrated is to stay away from diuretics. Some medications are diuretics. Also, coffee is a diuretic. Soda can also have the same effect. Instead of coffee, drink tea. Tea is just some leaves and lots of water. I'll go into tea drinking later in the book. It's fascinating.

Instead of drinking sugar-laden and caffeinated soda, drink seltzer water. Seltzer has no calories and gives you that bubbly soda feeling. There are many flavors you can choose from. The one that comes closest to drinking soda is black cherry. Although there are no sweeteners, it does rather have a sweet taste to it.

My favorite drink is plain seltzer with freshly squeezed lime. This taste is so refreshing on a hot summer day. This does more for me than a can of Coke.

If you are still craving a sweet drink, you can mix seltzer with orange juice or apple juice. As mentioned earlier, another favorite drink is to mix Ginger Kombucha and seltzer. This is a great way to satisfy a sugar craving and stay hydrated. Kombucha tastes sweet but is low in sugar.

Fruits

Another way to stay hydrated is with fruit. As you can guess, watermelon is a great way to get fluids into your body. However, all fruits and vegetables have water in them. Have you ever seen a carrot go through a juicer? You would think a carrot is solid with no water content. But if you watch a carrot go through a juicer, you will see a lot of juice come out.

Instead of having snacks like potato chips or crackers, you should eat carrots and other vegetables. I often make a snack out of baby carrots and radishes. I cover them with salt and pepper. If you are someone who is accustomed to potato chips and other dry snacks, this may sound unappetizing. Over time, you will get used to it. You will no longer have a desire for dry snacks.

Don't forget, most people are dehydrated. One of the first things they do when you enter the emergency room is hook you up to an IV to get fluids into your body.

When I got my viral infection that kicked off my whole heart palpitation problem, I was put on an IV. Sometimes they have vitamins and minerals in there. For the most part, it's to get fluids directly into your system.

While I was lying there on the hospital bed, I didn't feel much like drinking water. In fact, it probably would have made me throw up because I was feeling quite nauseous. Getting fluids intravenously was a strange feeling because I was in the hospital bed for about half an hour, and I didn't have anything to drink, but all of a sudden, I had to pee like a racehorse.

After lying in the hospital bed for another half hour, I had to go again. At first, I could not figure it out. I said to myself, "I didn't drink anything." Then I realized all those fluids in my IV were working their way to my bladder. Who knows? I didn't.

Full belly

This one, I'm reasonably sure you may not have heard of. I only learned about it by experiencing it and then researching it.

The theory about the full belly is that when your stomach is full, it puts pressure on your vagus nerve. Your vagus nerve runs from your brain stem all the way through your belly. Your vagus nerve is responsible for your parasympathetic nervous system. This is the nervous system that keeps you calm. Your sympathetic nervous system puts you in fight or flight mode. Some people call this fight, flight, or freeze mode.

When your vagus gets pressure from your full belly, it doesn't operate very well, and your sympathetic nervous system takes over. That's what gives you heart palpitations.

My personal experience has been that if I stuff myself, I could count on some kind of erratic heart activity. Unlike the other triggers mentioned, I rarely experienced a full-on heart palpitation. Well, at least if I just drink enough water.

Full-blown episode

There was one time that I had a full-blown heart episode where I thought I was going to die. It was actually my first full-blown tachycardia episode. I was at my father's house, cleaning out his attic. During a break, I went to Wendy's and got a double bacon cheeseburger, Dr. Pepper, and French fries. Yeah, I don't eat that crap today. Back then, I didn't eat so well. I was at least twenty to thirty pounds heavier then.

Anyway, when I brought the whole mess home from Wendy's, I scarfed it down in no less than three minutes. I was hungry. I wolfed down the burger. Then the highly salted fries kept getting inserted into my mouth like candies on a conveyor belt. Then it all got washed down with a sugar-laden and highly caffeinated Dr. Pepper. To top it off, I stuffed myself to the gills. This was a heart palpitation bomb in the making. My belly was full. I could barely walk.

Anyway, I continued to move boxes out of the attic. Then Bam! My heart goes racing at 200 beats per minute. This was the first time this happened to me, so I just thought this was clogged arteries and a good old-fashioned heart attack taking place.

The house was empty, and no one knew I was there. I didn't have my phone with me, so I couldn't call an ambulance. I figured I would go outside and stand in my driveway. If I collapsed, someone would see me.

I stood in my driveway, clutching my chest, waiting for the lights to go out. I could feel the blood squishing through my body. My heart was just pounding away. I could hear it in my head. Bump, bump. Bump, bump. I felt like I was hearing an audio track from a movie about a character who is about to be caught committing a murder.

Almost as quickly as my heart started to pound at 200 beats per minute, it regained a normal rhythm. What a relief!

I stood there and said, "What the hell was that?"

First, I attributed my episode to the double bacon cheeseburger. It seems like the right culprit. Later, when I found out about caffeine and sugar being triggers for heart palpitations, I blamed my episode on the burger *and* Dr. Pepper. Then, when I learned more about triggers, I realized that my full belly also played a role.

This was definitely a combination of a good heart episode. Let's see what was going on here. I ate a fattening burger (probably loaded with preservatives and salt). That is bound to clog some arteries and keep my heart working hard to keep the blood flowing. Then the massively salted fries probably constricted my arteries or whatever it is that salt does. Then I had a nice dose of caffeine. Then to top it off, I had a nice dose of sugar. It is incredible people don't die left and right from this combination. It just goes to show how resilient we are to the crap we put into our bodies.

Needless to say, I do not ever eat that kind of food anymore. I no longer consume caffeine. My sugar intake is minimal. I eat burgers, but often I just eat half of the burger and take the rest home. This eases the pressure on my belly.

Have you seen the burgers that they serve at these casual restaurants? They're huge! Probably 800 calories or more. Just for the burger. Forget about the fries and everything else.

Other than gulping water, I'm cautious about stuffing my belly to the brim.

Eating too fast

This is closely related to overeating and having a full belly. However, even if I don't stuff myself, if I eat too fast, sometimes my heart would jump a little bit.

If I eat chips or nuts and I eat them too fast, I definitely feel it.

Eating slow helps you to digest food. The saliva in your mouth is part of the digestive process. Some medical professionals suggest chewing your food at least twenty or more times before swallowing. They advocate masticating your food into a liquid before swallowing.

I think that is a little extreme. However, I am practicing eating slowly and chewing my food ten or more times. I haven't felt any significant benefits from the super slow way of eating. Like I said earlier, I had definitely felt my heart bumping around whenever I ate extremely fast.

Scary movies/Disturbing scenes

Here is another unlikely trigger. You may not have experienced it or have but just didn't realize it. I first discovered this when I was close to being 75% cured. I had been feeling good for days. I had not had any heart palpitations for about a week. I had been doing all the right things. I had been eating well and treating my body well.

After feeling good for about a week, I watched a movie about knights and medieval Europe. Have you seen Braveheart? Kind of like that. Except this movie was a lot more graphic. Do you remember the scene in Braveheart where Mel Gibson's character (William Wallace) gets eviscerated by that evil executioner? In Braveheart, they didn't show you the gory details. They just leave it up to you to imagine what was going on.

However, in the movie that I was watching, they didn't do that. Through the magic of special effects, they showed a man disemboweled while he was being hanged. They showed his guts falling out of his body. I was so disturbed by the realism of this scene that my heart started to go into an episode of rapid and erratic heartbeats.

It took me a few minutes to calm down.

If this was the only incident with scary movies and disturbing scenes, I might have brushed it off. But after that moment, I started to recall the other times where my heart was triggered.

I used to watch "fail" videos on YouTube, where people often fell on their heads after trying some crazy stunt. Usually, I would close my eyes. Not one particular scene really set me off. But the many scenes built up in my mind had a significant effect on my condition. We will discuss that later in the book.

Lack of sleep

This trigger is not something most people would notice right away, but it's definitely a major trigger for those who suffer from heart palpitations.

Whenever I don't get enough sleep, I definitely feel it.

Part of the reason I don't get enough sleep is because I get insomnia in the middle of the night. Going to bed and getting to sleep at 9:00 is not a problem. It's just when I wake up at

2:15 to go to the bathroom. I never fall back to sleep. I end up with only about five hours of sleep.

When I lack sleep, I can really feel it in my chest. I feel a flutter that will not go away. If combined with another trigger (such as watching a disturbing scene in a movie), then it will definitely set me off.

Bending over

This is one trigger I hear a lot from people who aren't really sure what kind of problem they have. They just report that they were bending over to pick up a child or taking a full trash bag out of a trash can, and then they get these heart palpitations. Or some people reported getting a rapid heartbeat while doing their laundry and taking clothes out of the dryer.

I thought nothing of these people because I never experienced anything like what they were describing. Until one day I was at the gym. I had a massive SVT episode, and it was while I was bending over. I was not completely bent over because I wasn't on my feet. I was sitting on a yoga mat doing some stretches. I was stretching my groin and hamstring muscles. While I was on the mat, I was reaching for my toes with my nose was touching my knees.

That's when it hit me. My heart was beating at two hundred beats a minute. I was clutching my chest and breathing heavily.

What I noticed after this memorable incident is that my attacks seem to come when I'm at rest. This seems to be common for many people. Before my SVT episode, I had been lifting weights and running on a treadmill, and nothing happened. Once I slowed down and rested my body, that's when it hit me. Unfortunately, I have no explanation for this—nor did I find anything during my research into this.

Now, I just employ a simple trick that has helped me avoid many incidents. Whenever I bend over to get something, I breathe out and hold my breath for five to ten seconds. I will explain this more in a later chapter. But for now, it works every time.

Summary

These are just a few triggers that I have succumbed to. The biggest thing for me is the combination of triggers such as sugar and caffeine or caffeine and alcohol or sugar, and alcohol.

Many of these you may be aware of, but many you may not be aware of at all. Eliminating these triggers got me to be about 65% cured of my heart palpitations. It took a combination of eliminated triggers and adding supplements that brought me closer to 75% cured. We will explore vitamins and minerals in the next chapter.

Key takeaways:

- The biggest triggers are sugar, caffeine, and alcohol
- Bending over is a common trigger for some people

- Breathing out and holding the breath for ten seconds may alleviate the onset of a heart event

- MSG and sweeteners often hidden in everyday foods can be triggers for many people

- Staying hydrated with fruit and vegetables is an excellent way to alleviate heart events

-3-

Vitamins and Minerals

Before discovering a host of triggers, I actually researched and found some supplements that were going to help me. Like most people, I wanted a pill. I didn't want someone (like a doctor) to tell me to do without something. I didn't want to be told I had to give up caffeine. I wanted a pill. I didn't want to be told to give up sugar. I wanted a pill. I didn't want someone to ask me to give up alcohol. I wanted a pill. I didn't want someone to tell me...well, you get the idea. I wanted a pill, damn it!

We've been brainwashed in our medicine-abundant society to find a pill to cure our ills. As you will discover by reading this entire book, this is not the way to go. However, it's an excellent place to start. That's what this chapter is all about.

Magnesium

After my doctor told me my heart palpitations were all in my head a few times, it started to wear off. I no longer was able to go six months on just thinking that it was all in my head. I was getting heart palpitations more and more frequently.

Since I had major heart palpitations after my viral infection, I was on the hunt for something to ingest that would relieve me of my pain and discomfort.

The first thing I found was magnesium. You may have discovered this, too. My first foray into the world of magnesium was magnesium oxide, which is the most popular form sold in stores like CVS and Walgreen's. If you haven't heard of either one of these pharmacies, then you are definitely in some parts of the country or world that I've never been to.

When I first took my first dose of magnesium, it was a dream come true. The magnesium seemed to have cured my problem right away. I took magnesium for a few weeks with excellent results.

When I learned of my good results, I wanted to find out more about this magnesium and how it was so effective. This, I learned, was somewhat of a mistake. A recurring theme in my journey was that I was giving these things (triggers, supplements, foods, etc.) too much thought. I was researching too much. If you do enough research, you will end up questioning everything. One day, eggs are good for you. The next day, they are bad for you.

This happened with magnesium and me. It wasn't that anyone said magnesium was terrible. In fact, everyone was saying that it was good. The problem was everyone had a different opinion as to what kind of magnesium was the best. There are at least half a dozen different types of magnesium, and everyone has a view on every one of them. Everyone agrees that magnesium oxide is the most inferior form of magnesium. As soon I read that, guess what happened? It stopped working.

When I found out about the side effects of magnesium, guess what happened? I had extended stays in my bathroom. For those who don't know (and maybe I shouldn't tell, but I'm gonna anyway), magnesium oxide (and other forms) have a laxative effect. Ever heard of Milk of Magnesia? Well, that's magnesium—the kind that lets your bowels loose. Fun, right?

Research

I was doing more research because I heard that some were better than others—in terms of bathroom action. Unfortunately, not many people came out and said which one was the best. They all hinted at it and claimed that magnesium oxide was the worst. They said things like, "Some are better than others, but magnesium oxide is the worst." Gee, thanks. That was a big help. Not really.

After trial and error on a few of them, I finally settled on *Doctor's Best,* which is magnesium glycinate. I would tell you about the other ones, but I forgot which ones they were. Everyone has a different experience, so the best thing I can say is to experiment. Just don't experiment while camping in the woods—if you get my drift.

This form of magnesium (glycinate) seems to work well for me. However, I must spread out the dose throughout the day. For instance, on the package, it says, "take two tablets twice daily." I only take one tablet twice daily or even only one a day. Now, I don't take much at all.

Science

Here's a little science behind magnesium. Magnesium relaxes your muscles, and calcium contracts your muscles. Guess what? Your heart is a muscle. You knew that already, but I'm just reminding you.

Anyway, you need magnesium to help with heart function. The problem is that most people are overloaded with calcium because the crooked milk industry has been telling us that we need more and more calcium. This is not true at all.

I won't go into all the science here. Calcium supplements are terrible for you. You don't need this much calcium. You already get enough in your diet. Look this up and do some research into this. Don't take my word for it. I'm just writing this based on memory. Anyway, many of us are overloaded with calcium.

I was too. So, when I started magnesium supplements, it really helped. In fact, I significantly reduced my calcium intake. Remember all that ice cream I stopped eating? No more ice cream. Remember when I stopped eating eggs for breakfast? No more calcium. Remember all that cereal I ate? No more calcium-laden milk. I do use almond milk in my hot cereal. I never took a supplement, so that didn't count.

Dr. Carolyn Dean

Much of what I learned about magnesium came from Dr. Carolyn Dean. I read her book, The *Magnesium Miracle*. If you want to know a lot about magnesium, this is a great book to read. Everything you ever wanted to know about magnesium is in that book.

This also brings to the point of magnesium and bathroom activities. There are many types of magnesium that people claim don't give you any bathroom activities. However, everybody is different, so it's hard to say.

However, Dr. Carolyn Dean has her own line of products that are supposed to help in this matter. One of her products is ReMag, which "has the highest known concentration of any magnesium." This is supposed to assist in the bathroom department. Quite frankly, I didn't notice much of a difference—both in terms of having fewer bathroom visits and helping my heart palpitations.

I'm not saying it won't help you. I just couldn't tell if it was helping me. It wasn't the miracle that I was looking for at the time. When I started using this product, I was far from cured. I was still having horrible heart palpitations. Hundred times a day. It was driving me nuts. I'm sure you know the feeling. So, I think it was not the right product at that time. I had a very frustrating attitude about my condition.

One final note: Dr. Carolyn Dean has high ratings on Amazon for both her books and her products. I definitely recommend that you read one of her books. It helps to be well educated on these matters—through books by ONE author, not a bunch of blog posts.

Transdermal magnesium

Believe it or not, you can take magnesium transdermally. This means that it soaks through your skin. It comes in the form of a spray. It is traditionally called magnesium oil, but it's not really an oil. It just feels oily when it makes contact with your skin. One of the brands I've tried is Ancient Minerals. Dr. Mark Sicus is a big proponent of transdermal magnesium. He has a bunch of videos on YouTube. Look him up and watch his videos.

Taurine

This was a supplement that someone on Amazon said helped them a lot with their heart palpitations. I tried it. It did help me a lot. However, after a few weeks, it wore off.

This seems to be a pattern for me. I would try something and think it's the miracle I've been looking for, and then it wears off. I guess it's the placebo effect in action. This is why, later in the book, I talk about the pros and cons of doing your research.

Taurine was definitely something I had hoped would work for me. I still take it for other issues and good health, but I'm not so sure how well it helped me with my heart palpitations. However, later in the book, I will discuss the placebo effect and how it will help you get your issues resolved.

Hawthorn Berries

In my opinion, this is one of the best supplements you can take for your heart palpitations. For me, it took me from 25% cured to about 75% cured. This is even better than magnesium.

I haven't discovered any known side effects with me or anyone else. However, there was a period I was taking massive doses (with other supplements), and my heart felt like it was slow.

Now, I only take 1 dose (565mg) a day. Some days, I don't even take it at all.

Also, there is a Hawthorn Berries tea that you can drink. I drink this from time to time. It's pretty good—that is if you like herbal teas.

L-Theanine

This was another supplement that someone on Amazon recommended. So far, it has worked out well for me. I use it if I want to have a good night's sleep. Sometimes if I'm out drinking, I will get an adrenaline rush, and my heart will start beating pretty fast. Not the SVT kind of fast, but more like I'm running or exercising. This supplement keeps me calm and helps me sleep. I just pop one of these and magnesium when I go to bed. I usually sleep through the night without any incident.

Basically, L-Theanine is derived from green tea. You would think it would have a caffeine effect, but it doesn't. L-Theanine actually calms you. That's why it is so good for your heart palpitations.

So far, I haven't had any side effects from taking this. However, everyone is different.

L-Arginine

This is another supplement that someone recommended on an Amazon review of a book about heart palpitations.

I started taking this supplement, and it has helped me a lot. Some people didn't feel anything. For me, it has been helpful. It's not the miracle cure I'd been searching for, but it still helps.

As you will see in this book, you will have to take and do a combination of things to cure your heart palpitations. Many of these things I still do on occasion. Also, a lot of them I just needed to get me to the next level.

You have to understand that your body is probably lacking a lot of vitamins and minerals. In the Western World, our diets are very poor and lacking in vital nutrients. Foods today don't have all the vitamins and minerals they once had. Fruit, vegetables, and meat are raised to look and taste good and increase crop yields. They are not raised to have high nutrition content. Providing enough vitamins and minerals doesn't factor in at all in the growing process.

Therefore, your body is severely lacking. This is why I believe many of these vitamins and minerals worked great for me and then tapered off. I still think they all played a role in getting me 97% cured. However, none of them by themselves is a miracle cure.

With that said, many of these vitamins and minerals did help with my overall health, so I'm happy about that.

Probiotics

During my journey to my 97% cure, I read a lot about the microbiome, which is your gut. Many health practitioners say this is where many of our problems lay. Some even say that if your gut flora is out of whack, then you could suffer from heart palpitations.

Let me point out here that many practitioners of all sorts of disciplines make the same claims of cures. I'm not saying they're wrong, but they are often not right—at least in my case.

Since magnesium gave me so much bathroom activity, I believed I may have flushed out much of my gut flora. In fact, even after I stopped taking magnesium, I was still depositing Carvel® soft-serve ice cream into the toilet. It took me a long time to get over it. I will tell you how I did it below.

Anyway, I tried probiotics to clean up my gut flora. As stated, I did this to replace what I may have lost during my era of magnesium (which was about three years). At first, the probiotics seemed to have worked. No more soft-serve ice cream! I was elated. I was dropping pebbles! I was so excited. But that only lasted two weeks. As mentioned before, this became a recurring theme. Everything I tried lasted two weeks, but then I was back to where I started.

Not precisely to where I started but close enough to bum me out. Again, I must emphasize that every little step counts toward the ultimate goal, no matter how much it may seem otherwise. I wish someone had told me that. Instead, I would just get upset that something wasn't working. This obviously didn't help me at all.

Anyway, I was back to serving up soft-serve ice cream, so I needed to find something that was going to help me with the fallout of overdosing on magnesium. I really needed to clean up my gut flora.

Daily fiber

All the books about the microbiome talked about getting enough fiber. I had a hard time believing I wasn't getting enough fiber. I was eating lots of fruits and vegetables. By this time, my diet consisted mostly of plants. In fact, I ate entirely plant-based meals Monday through Friday. On the weekends, I would have dinners with some kind of meat.

As you may or may not know, meat has no fiber. Bread and grains have some fiber. But fruit and vegetables have the most fiber.

Anyway, I decided to take daily fiber in the form of a supplement. I'm sure you've heard of FiberCon™ or Metamucil™. I was taking some store-brand pills. This is supposed to "keep you regular"—whatever that means.

Guess what?

It worked! No more Carvel® soft-serve ice cream! Hello, Dippin' Dots®! I felt like a deer out in the woods. It was Heaven. My gut flora had been restored. I was so happy. So very happy...until...

...my bathroom issues came back. Ugh! Hi, Carvel® soft-serve ice cream. Goodbye, Dippin' Dots®. Sad face. Sad face.

This was a low point in my life. I really felt like I solved my bathroom issues. But I hadn't. I tried nearly everything.

pH water drops

I heard about pH water drops in a book about curing heart palpitations. A big shout-out goes to Nick Walsh (Morgan Adams), author of *7 Proven Methods to Safely Prevent Heart Palpitations!*

Like everything else I heard about solving my heart palpitations problem, I decided to give pH water drops a try. Basically, you squirt six drops into your glass of water, and your water will have the proper pH balance.

The kind I use is called pH Booster Drops from AlkaBoost™. They're not that expensive, and you can get them on Amazon.

However, these didn't seem to have any effect on my heart palpitations. I still felt the same. There was one good side effect...

Can we say good-bye Carvel® soft-serve ice cream and hello Dippin' Dots®? This was the miracle I was looking for. I mean, in terms of my bathroom activities. It wasn't a miracle for my heart condition. But it did clear up my bathroom escapades once and for all. And I really do mean "once." Because after only one dose (6 drops in 8 ounces of water), my situation was all cleared up. It was amazing. I still use the pH drops because I figure, "Why not?"

B complex

Someone on YouTube suggested that heart palpitations were caused by a lack of B vitamins. (As you can probably tell, I get a lot of medical advice from YouTube and Amazon versus going to a real doctor. As mentioned, real doctors were no help to me. You may have experienced this yourself).

Anyway, this YouTuber (he was not a doctor) suggested getting more B vitamins into my diet. He said we are just not getting enough B vitamins in our diets.

He recommended beef livers. I couldn't find any beef livers. I looked out the window and then on Amazon. After that, I gave up and said, "Damn it, just give me a pill."

So, that's what I did. I got some B-complex vitamins at Trader Joe's.

They work! I was thrilled with the results. My heart palpitations reduced a little more. I was pleased about that.

The only problem with B-complex vitamins, or rather taking the advice of ingesting B-complex vitamins, is that every manufacturer has a different formulation. On Trader Joes' container, it has Niacin (b), Vitamin b6, Folate (b), b-12, and a bunch of other stuff.

Other manufacturers will have something completely different and call it B-complex. I guess what I am saying is that you will have to go and experiment.

Anyway, these B vitamins brought me closer to my goal of being cured. I would say, at this point, I was about 78% cured.

Vitamin D + Vitamin K

I learned about vitamin D through another issue I was having at the time. Since my heart palpitations were so bad, I stopped working out hard at the gym. I actually went to the gym with a doughnut, sat on the sofa, and watched everyone else work out. Therefore, I started to become very sedentary.

With this, my calves were cramping up like crazy. I was getting anxious because a friend of mine had deep vein thrombosis (DVT). This is basically a blood clot in your deep vein. One of the signs or symptoms is stiff and sore calves.

I thought about going to a doctor because this seemed like a real problem that many people had. But before going to a doctor to have my legs scanned or whatever it is they do, I decided to do some research online about stiff calves.

During my research, I found out about Vitamin D. I read a book that basically said we, people in the Western World, are woefully lacking vitamin D. We don't get enough sun, and there are no foods that provide vitamin D.

In fact, vitamin D isn't even a vitamin. It's a hormone that your body makes when it is exposed to the sun. With all the sun scares this country has had over the years, nobody is getting much sun. Everyone is slathering sunscreen all over their bodies—thereby preventing the sun's rays from penetrating our skin. And guess what? No vitamin D.

Again, modern medicine has done us wonders. Give it enough time, and the medical community will say, "Oh, do you remember when we told you to stay out of the sun and to slather sunscreen all over your bodies? Yeah, well, that was a mistake. In fact, it's the sunscreen that you are slathering all over your body that's causing skin cancer. You see, it really doesn't make sense that the sun—our life essence—would poison us. So, you see, it was all bullshit. Go back to enjoying the sun."

But now, we're stuck with all the misinformation about vitamin D and sunscreen.

To top it all off, the recommendations that the medical community provides are entirely inadequate. They say you should get anywhere between 400IU to 800IU a day. I take anywhere from 5,000IU to 10,000IU a day and feel great. In fact, if I don't take 10,000IU a day, my legs cramp up.

Have you heard of rickets? That's caused by a vitamin D deficiency.

This book is much too short, and I'm much too uneducated to go into depth about vitamin D, but I suggest you look into this.

As far as helping with heart palpitations, I think vitamin D has been beneficial to me. However, that's just me. I haven't read any studies or read anyone else having the same experience. Again, this book is about my experience, so I just wanted to pass this along.

By the way, if you do take large doses of vitamin D, you should take vitamin K with it as well. It's best to research this on your own.

Summary

I introduce you to some vitamins and minerals that have been very helpful to me. As I will mention later in the book, the big three are magnesium, Hawthorn Berries, and L-Theanine. I didn't take B-complex until then, but I think it was beneficial to me. While vitamin D was taken for another reason, I feel it also had a positive effect on getting me closer to my 97% cure.

Key takeaways:

- Big 3 supplements are magnesium, Hawthorn Berries, and L-Theanine
- B-complex is a supplement that is worth exploring more
- pH water drops did wonders for my bathroom activities
- A clean gut will help with your heart palpitations

-4-

Foods

What you put into your body has a significant effect on how your heart functions. Eat the wrong foods, and your heart is not going to be happy. Eat the right foods, and you are on your way to a more joyful heart.

In this chapter, we will explore the foods I discovered that helped me get over my heart palpitations. As a reminder, these are the only foods that I found to be helpful. Many other foods can be beneficial to you.

You must explore them for yourself, but at least you know what foods a fellow sufferer recommends. Let's get started.

Magnesium-rich foods

While I was on my magnesium kick, I was looking for natural forms of magnesium. I didn't want to visit the poop station too much, so taking a lot of magnesium supplements was out.

Fortunately for me, many of the foods that I enjoyed already had a healthy dose of magnesium. Here are the top foods for magnesium:

- Dark chocolate
- Avocados
- Nuts/Almonds
- Seeds
- Whole grains
- Bananas
- Leafy greens
- Black beans
- Pumpkins seeds
- Molasses

Although these foods are known to have the highest concentration of magnesium, I didn't see a benefit from eating these foods versus taking a supplement. Granted, these foods do have a lower concentration of magnesium than a pill. However, I was eating a lot of this stuff and didn't see a huge difference.

I still eat these foods, but I don't rely on them to give me a magnesium boost. Also, I was eating a lot of potassium-rich foods, such as potatoes. But that didn't help with my heart palpitations. However, eating a potato for breakfast was a lot better than eating a bowl of cereal or a greasy egg.

While I didn't notice a huge or immediate difference with these foods, I think consuming these was a lot better than the alternatives. Having a ripe banana in my oatmeal is better than table sugar. Having an avocado on my salad is better than chicken on my salad. Having nuts and almonds is better than potato chips as a snack.

Mineral water

Mineral water is precisely what it sounds like. It's water with mineral content. I say "mineral content" instead of "*high* mineral content" because most of the mineral water you see in the grocery store does not have a significant amount of minerals in the water. In fact, it says it right there on a bottle of S.Pellegrino®.

Not a lot of mineral waters that claim to be mineral water have many minerals in them. I was looking for water that had a lot of magnesium in it. The beauty of this is that it is natural magnesium. It comes from a river that is rich in minerals.

One brand that I was able to find in grocery stores is Gerolsteiner®. It's from Germany. I haven't seen it everywhere, but Whole Foods sells it.

Here is the mineral content of their water:

- pH   5.9 to 6.0
- Bromine (Br)   0.12
- Calcium (Ca)   348
- Chloride (Cl)   39.7
- Bicarbonate (HCO_3)   1816
- Fluoride (F)   0.21
- Lithium (Li)   0.13
- Manganese (Mn)   0.39
- Magnesium (Mg)   108
- Nitrate (NO_3)   5.1

- Potassium (K)   10.8
- Silica (SiO2)   40.2
- Sodium (Na)   118
- Strontium (Sr)   2.9
- Sulfate (SO4)   38.3

So, did this water work for me?

It sure did!

My heart felt so much better after drinking this water. At the height of my heart problems, I drank about sixteen ounces of this a day.

Here is a quote from an Amazon customer that reflects my sentiments precisely:

> *"The high magnesium content is the most of any mineral available, and it has helped raise my magnesium level when medication and food couldn't. I feel so much more energetic because of this water."*
> –Jake S.

I highly recommend drinking this water. It was a lifesaver for me when I was at my wit's end trying to figure what to do about my crazy heart palpitations.

Tea

I touched upon this before in an earlier chapter, but I want to expand on this further because this has been very important to me.

Before drinking tea, I drank a lot of coffee. Compared to some people, probably not so much. But I would go to Starbucks or Dunkin' Donuts twice a day and get a medium coffee. I would load it with cream and sugar.

I thought nothing of it at the time. Coffee just seemed normal to me. Have some caffeine and have some fun. Why not, right? I drank it in the morning before going to the gym. I would drink it in the evening before going to a tennis match.

But since my bout with heart palpitations, I had to give it all up. Coffee, with its caffeine and sugar content, really is a big trigger when it comes to heart palpitations.

So, this brings me to drinking tea.

Actually, not so fast.

For me to give up coffee, I had to go through a lot of effort. First, I started drinking decaf coffee to lower my caffeine intake. Then I started drinking less and less. But I couldn't give it up. I loved it so much.

Did you know that a latte is just like coffee ice cream? It's true. It's got cream and sugar, just like ice cream.

When I started to realize that coffee was just like ice cream, I began to realize how silly it was to be drinking coffee before going to work. I should just have some ice cream instead. How does that sound? You're going into the office with an ice cream cone instead of a latte. Think about that for a moment.

I had a hard time giving up coffee. I really tried. Even though I was aware that it was a trigger for me, I still had a hard time giving it up.

Around this time, I went to see a hypnotherapist to help me with my coffee addiction. She didn't seem to help me much. However, there was something that she said that made me switch to drinking tea. She said that I probably liked coffee because of the hot liquid going down my throat. I didn't realize it at the time, but she was right.

So, I started to drink tea.

My first foray into the kingdom of tea was when I went to Panera Bread®. I filled my cup with hot water, and I tossed in a tea bag. I drank it straight up. I didn't put any milk or sugar in it. I figure that would defeat the purpose of my whole mission of trying to give up a bad trigger.

The tea I drink is Ginger Peach. It is a light herbal tea. I tried hard to make it a habit, so I went back to Panera Bread® the next morning and got my tea. I repeated this over and over.

Occasionally, I had a powerful craving for coffee, so I let myself have a decaf. However, I would pay for it later. On one particular day, I was driving to work with my coffee in hand without a care in the world. At this point, I was having irregular heart palpitations, so I didn't know that this coffee indulgence would trigger one. But it did. Massively. Fortunately, I was on a slow country road. I pulled over to the side of the road and waited to die. Because that's how I felt. My heart was going crazy. It was banging all over the place.

Anyway, back to the tea drinking. After several months, I realized how silly it was to pay more than three or four dollars for some hot water and a tea bag. So, I bought an electric kettle to make hot water at home. It was easier and faster than putting a pot on the stove. It wasn't nearly as complicated as making coffee at home: just some hot water and a tea bag.

Since I was used to my Ginger Peach tea from Panera Bread®, I bought the same brand at Whole Foods. The beautiful thing about tea is that there is so much variety. Coffee has a few types but not as many as tea.

Quit coffee

I strongly urge you to quit coffee and start drinking tea. As discussed before, if you drink coffee with cream and sugar, you're just eating ice cream. Would you give ice cream to your children two or three times a day? Think about that.

If you're one of the crazy people who drink your coffee black, then you still have the caffeine issue. That is a significant trigger for people like us with heart palpitations.

By the way, the vast majority of tea that I drink is herbal tea, which means it has no caffeine. The Ginger Peach tea that I drink is a decaffeinated version. It's a black tea, but the other teas I drink are all herbal teas.

Sea salt

When I was reading books by Dr. Carolyn Dean, she recommended drinking water with a pinch of sea salt. Sea salt has many minerals that your regular table salt doesn't have.

The kind I use is HimalaSalt®, which is the brand name for pink Himalayan salt. I put a ½ teaspoon in hot water. Doing this also helped with my heart palpitations. It may have been a placebo effect, but I felt better. Besides, I like the taste of saltwater. I drink it almost every day. Sometimes I drink it more than once a day. For a while, I had an addiction, so I needed to lay off.

I generally use this pink sea salt in place of regular table salt. It doesn't have a strong taste like regular table salt, but you can still get used to it.

Onions

One day I made a fantastic discovery. One morning instead of my usual two fried eggs and red peppers, I decided to make a new dish. The dish I created was broccoli, mushrooms, and onions sautéed in a pan. It was delicious.

The fantastic thing is that it did wonders for my heart. Later, I discovered that the onions were the main ingredient that did wonders for my heart. Ever since then, I have tried to eat one whole onion every week.

Many places online back up my claim that onions are beneficial to the heart. But I don't need their endorsement because I felt the effects of eating onions. Onions are rich in B vitamins, including folate (B9) and pyridoxine (B6). They play vital roles in metabolism, red blood cell production, and nerve function.

Also, onions are a good source of potassium, which is also good for your heart. I've seen the benefits of potassium-rich foods firsthand.

Finally, onions have been shown to reduce cholesterol and lower inflammation. This is key to helping you feel healthy. As we will discuss later in the book, feeling fit is essential to getting to your cure. I know it has helped me tremendously.

Preparation

The best way I like to prepare onions is to fry them in a pan with a little oil. Sweet Vidalia onions are my favorite. As the name suggests, they have a sweet flavor when you cook them. They call this "caramelizing." And it's a good name for it because they do have that sweet flavor.

Sometimes I put these caramelized onions on top of my baked potatoes. By the way, the best potatoes to eat are Yukon Gold potatoes. They have a buttery look, texture, and taste. They are a lot better than white Russet potatoes. Anyway, adding caramelized onions adds a sweet flavor and moisture to my potatoes. Plus, I'm getting a real potassium punch.

As stated earlier, I make my "Broccoli Fry," which is broccoli, mushrooms, and onions. I use very little oil. This is delicious and makes an excellent breakfast. Sometimes I will throw in an egg or two.

I also use red onions in salads and sandwiches. You can eat red onions raw because they are not as strong as white or yellow onions.

I highly recommend that you get more onions in your diet. Onions have been one of the more significant contributors to getting me closer to a 97% cure.

Along with onions, you can eat shallots, garlic, and green onions.

Sweet potatoes

I call sweet potatoes my "magic energy." Whenever I eat sweet potatoes, I'm able to increase my energy and endurance. I first discovered sweet potatoes when I was very active in tennis. I would eat a sweet potato before a tennis match and feel like I was on fire.

Sweet potatoes played a role in my recovery. I don't know how. I don't have any scientific studies, but I know that my heart feels better when I have a sweet potato.

Preparation

Like all my other recipes, I like to keep things simple. I figure the simpler you make it, the easier you will stick to it. With sweet potatoes, I keep it really simple. You will see many recipes on YouTube where people cut them up, slather them with oil, and bake them in the oven. I don't do any of that. I keep it simple.

I nuke (microwave) a medium potato for two minutes to soften the insides. Then I dowse it in water before wrapping the potato in tin foil. Then I shove it in the oven for 47 minutes at 450 degrees.

When I yank it out of the oven, I peel away the skin. Unlike regular potatoes, sweet potato skins can be very tough and not very palatable. Therefore, I take off the skin. Then I put the potato in a bowl and mash it up. For extra creaminess, you can put it in a food processor. But like I said, I like to keep things simple. So, I mash it up with a fork.

At this point, your potato may seem a little dry. To moisten it up, you can add some butter. This is what I do. But I am always careful about how much butter I add, realizing that the more butter I add, the more fattening this sucker is gonna be. It's your choice. If you don't care about how fattening it is, then load it up with butter. The more butter you add, the better it tastes.

Microbiome

At this point—which was about 56% cured—I was looking for more ways to be 100% cured. I heard a lot about how important it is to keep the gut clean and free of crap. So, I studied quite a bit about the microbiome. I read a few books on the matter.

Some of it got pretty extreme—like a fecal matter transplant. A fecal matter transplant is taking someone else's shit and shoving it up your ass and into your inner sanctum. That sounded a little extreme to me. I wouldn't mind, however, if they put me to sleep and kept the donor's identity a secret.

Also, at this point, I was taking so much magnesium, I was having some nasty poops. I started to think my microbiome was all messed up.

Summary

Overall, I tried to keep my diet clean. I don't eat cereal with milk. I don't eat a lot of things that come out of a box. I eat plenty of fruits and vegetables. I drink tea, not coffee. I don't go out a lot, except for an excellent restaurant. In other words, I don't frequent fast food and casual dining establishments. They have a lot of preservatives and hormones in their foods.

Key takeaways:

- Magnesium-rich foods are helpful but not as potent as a supplement
- Mineral water with high mineral content like Gerolsteiner® from Germany can be beneficial
- Switch from coffee to herbal tea
- Onions were a huge help to me—eat one a week

-5-

Physical Remedies

Walking

Doing strenuous exercise at the gym was no longer an option for me. I could no longer run on a treadmill without my heart going haywire. I couldn't even lift weights without my heart skipping beats. I still wanted to go to the gym. It had become a daily routine that I had kept up for over thirty years. The idea of not exercising made me feel old and fat.

Instead of all the strenuous exercise, I just walked on the treadmill instead of jogging or running. It was difficult because even doing that little movement would make my heart go crazy. Heck, I couldn't even roll over in bed without my chest thrashing around.

The benefit of walking on the treadmill was that I read a lot about my heart condition. I would take my Kindle to the gym and prop it up on the treadmill dashboard. After an hour, I got a lot of reading in. I was able to read Dr. Carolyn Dean's books about magnesium plus books about other ways to overcome heart palpitations.

In some ways, I was almost grateful that I was forced to slow down. I just had to make the best of the situation.

Beach

When summer rolled around, I began walking on the beach in my hometown. It was a great alternative to the gym.

The salt air and sunshine helped me a lot. Also, walking barefoot helped me get in touch with the earth. I know it sounds woo-woo but walking barefoot really helped me feel connected to bigger things. It helped me keep my mind off my heart.

The woods

The most significant benefit I got from my walking routine was the discovery of walking in the woods. I had never been much of a hiker or a nature boy. I only hiked a few times in my youth, and that was it.

There was that time that I took a nature class at camp taught by a heavily bearded man by the name of Jerry. (Incidentally, this Jerry was a replica of Jerry Garcia of the Grateful Dead. Imagine that!) Anyway, I wanted to be more connected with nature.

This may have been the most significant turning point of my cure. When I was in the woods, I was able to see the wonder of nature. I will talk more about this in a later chapter, but I highly recommend you take time out of your day to walk in the woods. You will feel more connected, and you will soon think that your heart problem isn't as big as you think it is.

When you walk in the woods, you appreciate nature for what it is. Don't bring a phone or audio listening device. Don't bring a dog or anyone else. Just bring you.

Of all the remedies I've talked about so far or will talk about in later chapters, this is one of the more important ones. In our crazy rush, rush world, we forget about nature and the beauty it holds.

When I walk in the woods, I stop every few minutes and look up in awe at the trees and my surroundings. I will go more into depth about this in a later chapter, but you shouldn't overlook this one remedy.

Sunlight

Like most people, I spend (and spent) a lot of time indoors. This is very hazardous to your health. We aren't meant to spend this much time indoors and out of the sunlight.

The second year after my heart palpitations started, I made a concerted effort to go to the beach and spend a lot of time in the sunlight. Before my problem, I rarely went to the beach, even though it was only a ten-minute drive from my house. I only went a few times a month in the summer. I rarely got a tan.

I started to make an extra effort to sit in the sun. I'm glad I did because it helped me immensely. Like taking vitamin D, I felt so much better.

The funny thing is that the beach scared me because I had a major incident while swimming in the ocean. I would go to the beach, but I wouldn't go swimming. I was too scared.

Anyway, the sun did wonders for me and my heart. And I got a nice tan. Since I was able to work from home on many occasions, I took lunch breaks outside. When I did work at an office, I took many breaks outdoors to get some sun.

The best times to get sun is between 10:00 am and 2:00 pm. Although this is the time you are most likely to get burned, it's all the best time to get vitamin D. The secret is to spend fifteen minutes in the sun. The people who get burned spend hours in the sun during those prime sun-burning hours.

Since the sun is so intense during those hours, this activity makes it ideal for those who work in an office environment. All you need is fifteen minutes. The next time you sit at your desk with a bagel, try going outside for ten or fifteen minutes between 10:00 am and 2:00 pm. It will do wonders for you!

In addition to getting vitamin D, the sun also makes you feel alive and healthy. As discussed in later chapters, this is so important to your recovery. You can't just rely on pills and hope. Don't think you can only assault your heart with whatever remedy you choose. You must think in terms of overall health.

Standup Desk

Feeling healthy was one of the things that helped me through this process. The unhealthier I felt, the more my heart problem seemed to percolate. Sitting for ten hours a day didn't make me feel healthy. I felt fat, constricted, and frumpy.

6I work at home, so I purchased a standup desk for myself. This is one of the best investments I've made in recent years. It is an investment because the payoff has been tremendous. While using my standup desk, I feel more active and alive. I feel more aligned with my body. My spine feels straighter, too.

As I write this, I am standing up. For the first few months, I had to alternate between standing up and sitting down because my feet would hurt. My legs would also hurt. Also, I had trouble concentrating—such as writing the book you're reading now. Now, I can be at my standing desk all day long. I take short breaks and sit in a chair or sofa, but I no longer work in a sitting position. I'm able to concentrate just as much as if I was sitting.

Back brace

Since I was using the standup desk a lot and getting more aligned, I started to feel it in my back. So, I got a back brace. And wouldn't you know it, I felt a lot better in terms of my heart. With my back straighter, I felt more aligned and healthier.

This was key to my recovery: feeling healthy. The healthier I felt, the better. Vitamins and minerals were fine, but if I wasn't doing anything for my whole body, then it was no better than getting a pill from the doctor.

One thing I realized is that a heart palpitation is a symptom, not a disease. That's a crucial distinction. You can suppress symptoms with drugs and supplements. However, unless you address the underlying problem, you will always have the symptoms. My overall problem was that I was out of alignment, and I was unhealthy.

My back brace helped me feel more in alignment. I felt like I was doing something for my whole body rather than just trying to suppress my heart palpitations with supplements. If I only looked for remedies to control my heart palpitations, I would still have them today. It wasn't until I realized I had to treat my whole body, and that included my back.

Yoga

Yoga is also something I had never done until I had my heart palpitations. There is a part of me that believes that if I had practiced good health like my standup desk and yoga and many other healthy practices, I wouldn't have gotten any heart palpitations. On the other hand, I did visit the gym regularly, so I guess that theory is out. I was engaging in healthy activities.

Anyway, yoga helped me slow down and become in tune with my body. Also, it allowed me to overcome my fear of bending over.

The good thing about yoga was that I was able to exercise at home. This helped me to overcome many anxieties I had about going back to the gym after a major tachycardia episode.

Tai chi

Tai chi did many of the same things that yoga did for me. It allowed me to slow down. A lot of my heart issues came from me being wound up a lot. I had many hidden anxieties. Although I never had a panic attack (except for one ten-second episode in a grocery store), I believe I had some deeply rooted fears. Tai chi allowed me to go with the flow.

This helped me with my recovery because I was trying to find something that wasn't strenuous, like lifting weights or running. Walking on the treadmill was fine, but it didn't do anything for my strength and upper body.

Believe it, or not tai chi and yoga are strength exercises and help you build strength. They do this in a natural way, not some herky-jerky way that weightlifting does.

Stretching

Stretching allowed me to feel healthy and young. After getting my series of attacks, I didn't feel I could do all the heavy exercises. I was too scared. At this point in my troubles, I could barely climb the stairs without my heart beating more than a hundred beats per minute. It was agonizing. I'm sure you know the feeling.

I had to take one step at a time like a baby. On each level, I paused a moment before going on to the next step. At 48 years old, I felt like I was heading to an assisted living situation. It was awful.

Stretching helped me feel healthy. I felt like I was doing something for my body in a holistic way. Not being able to lift weights or run made me feel unhealthy. I felt like I was racing toward an early grave. Psychologically, it was debilitating.

However, as mentioned earlier, I had a significant tachycardia episode where my heart was beating at two hundred beats per minute. This freaked me out—then and for the next three weeks.

However, I had to get back on the horse and do my stretches as if nothing had happened. It wasn't easy. I was a little apprehensive. But I did it.

In the end, being able to do yoga and tai chi helped me overcome the anxieties I had about going back to the gym to get back to my regular routine. I like going to the gym versus staying home.

Sleep

This one is a biggie for me. Until recently, I didn't realize that I only needed 5 to 6 hours of sleep. The standard requirement is 7 to 8 hours of sleep. Through trial and error, I found out that I only needed five hours. However, not knowing this screwed me up because I kept trying to get eight hours of sleep. I would force myself to stay in bed. What ended up happening is I would get four hours or less.

I would go to bed earlier to catch up on sleep that I didn't get the night before. Then I would wake up in the middle of the night and not go back to sleep. I kept on trying to get eight hours. In the morning, I would lay in bed, trying to get my eight hours.

If I did get eight hours of sleep, I felt worse than if I only got five hours. I would feel tired and depressed. With only five or six hours, I felt energized.

I tell you this because everyone has a different requirement. Make sure you know exactly how many hours of sleep you need. Not knowing how many hours of sleep I needed set me back with my progress.

Once I figured out my sleep patterns, I felt better. I still have some sleep issues—like when I go out drinking or have caffeine. When I do have interrupted sleep, I get those little reminders I mentioned earlier. I know plenty of people who don't have any heart issues say that they get a bit of a restless heart if they don't get a good night's sleep. Sleep is essential to your heart. Make sure you get a good night's sleep!

Breathing

This was a big breakthrough for me. This got me to 88% cured.

You would think at the ripe old age that you are, you would know how to breathe by now. Right? However, many experts are telling us that we are breathing all the wrong way.

For starters, many people claim that deep breathing is terrible and that it activates the sympathetic nervous system. That's the one that causes a restless heart. From my experience and research, I agree with them.

Much of the deep breathing that yoga instructors tell you to do is wrong. Ancient texts on yoga talk about a different breathing pattern—not deep breathing.

I learned a lot about breathing from a book called *The Oxygen Advantage* by Patrick McKeown. This book opened my eyes to breathing and how it affects our health. This particular book is written for athletes and asthmatics. However, McKeown has written other books that are more in line with our problem of heart palpitations. One of them is *Anxiety Free*. I recommend you pick it up.

In these books, McKeown describes the Buteyko breathing method. Very briefly, Dr. Constantin Buteyko was a medical doctor in Russia. He noticed that severely unhealthy people breathed heavily and that they were primarily mouth breathers. They would breathe in and out and in again through their mouths.

Healthy people, on the other hand, breathe in and out, pause and in again through the nose. This is the typical breathing pattern for a healthy person. In McKeown's book, he has several breathing exercises you can use to practice your breathing. These exercises have helped me a lot. I strongly suggest that you read one of his books.

Tape over mouth

One simple thing that was a massive game-changer for me was putting tape over my mouth while sleeping. This forces you to breathe through your nose. The first night I did this, I immediately noticed a difference in my heart the following morning. My heart was calm, and I had very few heart palpitations throughout the day.

McKeown also has another book titled, *Close Your Mouth*. As the name suggests, you should breathe through your nose and not your mouth.

I could write nearly half the book on this topic alone. I want to keep things flowing, so I am keeping this section short. However, I do want to emphasize that this was one of the top three things I did to get me closer to my cure.

Although I should keep doing the breathing exercises during the day, I don't. I still tape my mouth shut at night. I'm just so used to it. Also, breathing through your nose is good for your overall health, not only your heart rhythms.

I won't rehash what other authors have talked about and written about. I do suggest you look up Buteyko breathing on Google, Amazon, and YouTube. I promise you that it will be a game-changer. It may not cure you, but it will significantly reduce your heart palpitations.

Breathing too much

Many activities will make you breathe a lot. One, of course, is rigorous exercise. Another is eating. Yes, eating. After you finish eating, you tend to breathe more. This is why whenever I had a full belly and I ate too fast, I would get mild palpitations.

Be aware of this the next time you eat a big meal. Are you eating too fast? Slow down! Chew slowly. Enjoy your meal and be mindful of what you are eating.

Breathe out and hold

Some of the breathing exercises include holding your breath. This is why I believe exhaling when bending over helps. When I think I'm about to have a tachycardia episode, I will breathe out forcefully and hold my breath for about ten or more seconds. This has helped me avoid a major heart palpitation event.

Once, I was in the grocery store, and an episode came out of nowhere. Normally, I would clutch my chest and maybe sit on the floor, thinking this was the big one. Now, I have a little trick that stops an attack in its tracks. Try it the next time you have a heart event. Just breathe out and hold.

It's important to breathe out and hold. Don't breathe in and hold. Also, don't exhale all the way out. Leave your lungs about one-third full. Don't hold your breath as if you're holding your breath underwater. You don't want to be out of breath when you start breathing again. You will end up breathing heavy still. That's what makes things worse. Hold your breath for about ten seconds or so until your attack passes.

Cold showers

I heard about this on YouTube. The theory on cold showers is that it soothes your vagus nerve. This nerve runs from your brain stem down to your gut. I tried this out for a while, and I did feel better. I've been taking cold showers for six months now. I started in the dead of winter when the temperatures were only in the single digits. That's cold. Nipply cold.

There is a strategy for taking cold showers. Many YouTubers say to jump in a cold shower and suck it up for as long as possible. That is not the way to go. For one, the ice-cold shower will have the opposite effect of what you are looking for.

You are using the cold shower to soothe your vagus nerve, which is responsible for "rest and digest." When you take an ice-cold shower but wish to get out as soon as possible, you are activating the "fight or flight" sympathetic nervous system. This could potentially make your condition worse.

What you want to do is start with a warm shower and, gradually, over time, turn the temperature down colder and colder. You want it to be cold enough to have the effect that you are looking for. You don't want the shower to be so cold that you want to jump out right away. I shoot for at least five minutes of really enjoying the shower.

I imagine myself outside in nature, taking a dip in a mountain stream on a beautiful sunny and hot summer day. That's about how cold you probably want your cold shower to be. You don't want your shower to be ice-cold—unless you can work up to that level comfortably.

Hot showers are very unnatural to the human body. There are very few natural hot bodies of water. Most bodies of water are rather cold—even in warmer climates. Most people wouldn't take a shower that is the same temperature as the water surrounding the Caribbean islands. Most people shower in water that is practically boiling. This is bad for your skin.

I found out that it's also bad for a person with heart palpitations. I had gone back and forth with hot and cold showers. There is no doubt in my mind that cold showers help with my fluttering heart. Whether it's the vagus nerve that's affected, I can't say for sure. What I do know is that cold showers work incredibly well for me—as long as they are not so cold that I want to jump out after ten seconds. I always shoot for five minutes. Even after five minutes, I want to stay in longer because it's so soothing.

Cold showers can be quite soothing once you get used to them. The trick is to go in slowly. I usually start with the temperature warm and then gradually turn the water colder.

Summary

While taking supplements is great for alleviating some of the strongest symptoms, you need to start taking care of your whole body. In this chapter, I discussed some modalities that have been extremely helpful to me in alleviating my heart palpitations.

When I couldn't do heavy lifting or run, I would walk on the treadmill and read a book. When the weather was beautiful, I would take walks on the beach. Through this whole process, I started to appreciate the outdoors and started taking walks in the woods. The vastness of the woods was very therapeutic for me.

Low-intensity exercises like yoga, stretching, and tai chi allowed me to keep up my strength without raising my heart rate too much. Keeping up with an exercise routine allowed me to get a good night's sleep. This is so very important to your overall health.

Since heavy exercises caused me to breathe heavy, I started practicing Buteyko breathing exercises so I could have a regular breathing pattern. Finally, I learned that taking cold showers is quite soothing to the vagus nerve. This nerve can affect your heart palpitations.

Key takeaways:

- Walking outside in the sun can be quite therapeutic
- Light exercises allow you to stay fit without setting off a heart event
- Learning how to breathe the correct way can be quite beneficial to your sympathetic and parasympathetic nervous systems
- Cold showers help soothe the vagus nerve

Section III
The Big Breakthrough

-6-

Psychology

What I discovered along my journey is that the condition I have or had is a lot more mental than I had initially thought. The reason why I was so focused on the physical was because of the massive onset of this condition came about after having a viral infection. After that, I've been trying to deal with my health through physical means.

I was reducing or removing triggers. I was taking supplements and changing my diet. I was exercising. But my most significant breakthrough was getting my head right.

I also had a hard time thinking this was a mental issue because I didn't have any of the usual anxiety and panic attack symptoms. Many people express a feeling of impending doom or that they cannot escape somewhere. Or that they are under a lot of stress at home or work.

My most significant attacks happened when none of those things happened. I was generally relaxed and in an excellent and confident mood. Naturally, I didn't think my problem with heart palpitations had anything to do with my mental state.

I had an easy life. I didn't have to work hard. Although I had a struggling freelance design and writing business, I had a comfortable life. I wasn't stressed. I don't have any kids, dogs, cats, birds, goldfish, or an ant farm, so no stress there. I had an easy life.

Yet, I was having the physical symptoms of a panic or anxiety attack, but I didn't feel any of the dread or impending doom that most people talk about when they have a panic attack. The only thing I felt at the actual point of having an attack of heart palpitations was that I was going to drop dead. However, this was after my attack had started, not before.

When I was stretching on a yoga mat and my attack happened, I was happy as can be. I didn't feel stressed. I felt relaxed. I was a little concerned about my heart since I had worked out heavily that day. However, I was still feeling pretty good when I had that major SVT while sitting and stretching on the floor.

When I had an attack while swimming in the ocean, I was happy as a clam. I had no fears or worries. I was having fun.

The numerous times I was driving around drinking coffee, I had no fears, worries, concerns, or stressors. Yet, I had massive attacks.

What was going on?

I didn't know. What I did know was that the remedies I talked about in this book were only working to a degree. They were suppressing my symptoms. I felt as if I was getting closer to resolving my issue once and for all.

But the key phrase here is "suppressing my symptoms." With all the techniques I've discussed so far, I was able to suppress my symptoms. My symptoms. It is not really resolving my underlying problem.

You see, these heart palpitations are a symptom of something bigger. It's your body telling you that your body is out of whack. In today's toxic society, most of us have bodies that are out of whack. Different people express different symptoms. Some people get obese; some get cancer; some get diabetes, and on and on.

The medical community calls these diseases, but they are symptoms of your body being out of whack. For us, it's heart palpitations. You can take vitamins and supplements to treat the symptoms. But just like any medication, once you stop taking the supplements, your symptoms will most likely come back. For some, they might need to get their magnesium back to optimal levels. But for most, we need to treat the underlying causes.

If you don't treat the underlying causes, then you will be taking supplements and other remedies forever. My goal was not to do that. I wanted to *cure* my problem. I didn't want to mollify the symptoms.

Even though I didn't have any outward signs of anxiety, I knew there was something deep down that was unresolved. I didn't know how to resolve it.

Meditation

I tried meditation (and still do it) for my heart palpitations. I believe it helped a little. Unfortunately for me, it wasn't anything significant. For you, it may be different. However, I still meditate today because it's good for overall mood adjustment.

I still recommend it for anyone who has heart palpitations.

If you haven't done any meditation, I would recommend listening to a guided meditation on YouTube or purchasing one on Amazon. There are millions of guided meditations on YouTube, so it doesn't make sense to buy one on Amazon.

The ones I started with are from *The Honest Guys*. Just do a search for them on YouTube or Google. They upload one video every day or something like that. I started with some of their ten-minute meditations. Then I moved up to twenty minutes and then finally, forty minutes.

Start slow. If you're going to do it on your own for the first time, then keep it simple. Just do one minute a day for a week. Then move up to five minutes, and so on.

Spiritual Journey

Recognizing that I have a nasty disposition and that I got myself into this mess, I started exploring a spiritual path.

I read books by Dr. Joe Dispenza, Michael Singer, and Wayne Dyer.

There are others that I haven't read, including Eckhart Tolle, Deepak Chopra, Alan Watts, and a bunch of others.

The one I latched onto the most was Dr. Joe Dispenza. He had a lot of science behind what he was teaching. I won't go into a lot of detail about him, but basically, he healed a major, paralyzing back injury just by thought alone.

He cured himself in ten weeks just by concentrating on healing his back. It's a pretty fantastic story. He's written the following books: *Becoming Supernatural*; *Breaking the Habit of Being Yourself*; *You Are the Placebo*, and *Evolve Your Brain*. I would recommend *Breaking the Habit of Being Yourself* and *You Are the Placebo*. I'm just starting to read *Becoming Supernatural*. However, *Evolve Your Brain* wasn't to my liking, so I don't recommend it.

I learned a lot about how the brain affects your body. This was a breakthrough for me. I won't go into details about what he teaches, but he also has guided meditations on his website. These have been incredibly helpful to me. They are truly amazing. The best thing is these audios are relatively cheap. I listen to them on my MP3 player in the quiet comfort of my home.

Michael Singer has a few books about letting things go. We keep so much bottled up but never let things go. We get angry at the stupidest things. Reading *Untethered Soul* helped me to relax about everything from work-related problems to traffic jams. Now, when things get tough, I just let things go.

Getting into this spiritual journey allowed me to see that my heart palpitations were not just a physical manifestation. Therefore, I cannot heal it only through physical means like supplements, breathing exercises, avoiding triggers, and so on. I needed to get my head right.

Walking in the woods

I mentioned walking on a treadmill at the gym earlier. That walking was a way of me getting exercise because I couldn't do any rigorous activities. The walking in the woods was for more my mind than my body. We will explore this later.

When I walk in the woods, I observe all that is around me. I appreciate all the trees, flora, and fauna. I appreciate the rocks, the streams, the dirt, and whatever else is in the woods.

I don't bring or use any electronic devices. I leave my MP3 player in the car, and I have my phone only for emergencies. Just in case, "I've fallen and can't get up." But I turn it off or put it in airplane mode. I forget I have it.

When I walk in the woods, I look at it in awe. No matter what time of year, I appreciate its grandeur. In the spring, I appreciate the bugs and insects. There is a clearing in the woods I call "the meadow." In the summer, I appreciate the thick canopy overhead.

In the fall, I love all the colors of the leaves. In the winter, I love the thick snow on the ground and the snow on all the branches. I love to see the footprints of other humans and the footprints of animals that often only come out at night. I even like to see some scat—as crazy as that sounds. Scat, by the way, is animal poop.

Having this appreciation for nature has helped me get into a very calm state. This, of course, helped with my recovery. When I first started walking in the woods, I had trouble walking up hills because my heart would start up and flutter. After three months, I was able to walk around, up and down, and climb over logs like a kid.

This was a big deal for me. It had been twenty years since I took a meaningful nature walk, and it had been three long years of debilitating heart palpitations. It was nice to see them go away. It was nice to know how my connection with nature helped me with my cure.

I can't stress enough how connecting with nature helped with my heart palpitations. Please do it as often as you can. You will feel so much better. I promise.

Gratitude journaling

Around this time, I was following several business development gurus. A lot of them and the spiritual gurus all suggest keeping and writing in a gratitude journal. In other words, every day, you should write down what you are grateful for.

This was new to me.

Usually, I would curse the world and all its problems. With the onset of my heart palpitations, I just cursed my heart. Being extremely angry at my heart and the world wasn't helping matters at all. Hard to believe, right?

I took to journaling very slowly. At first, I dabbled for a few days and then forgot about it for a few months. I just continued to bang my fist on my desk every time my heart started to act up. I was pent up. I wasn't grateful or appreciative of anything. I was angry because I couldn't figure out how to resolve my problem.

Doctors were of no help at all—as you probably may have experienced yourself. All they wanted to do was take my blood pressure and then give me a prescription for my blood pressure—which, by the way, only made my problem worse.

> Quick note: I didn't put anything in this book about taking medications because I never took any drugs for my heart palpitations. I've heard about all the side effects and all the bad stories. My advice is to stay away from medications. It's better to find a natural solution—like the ones you are reading in this book.

Anyway, after a few months of staggered, half-assed gratitude journaling, I started to go a little more hard-core. I would make three to eight entrees every day.

This helped me get into a calm state. I never realized how much negativity I allowed into my life and how much it affected my health. I will talk about this later in the book because it's a big topic.

Anyway, the best way to start journaling is to start. Start by saying, "I am grateful that it's a sunny day today." If it's raining, say, "I'm grateful that it's raining today because we need the rain. The rain makes all the flowers and trees so beautiful. I'm grateful that it was sunny yesterday."

Do you see how this works? You don't have to turn every seemingly negative thing into a positive. You don't have to say, "I'm thankful there was a lot of traffic today on the way home because I didn't want to eat my wife's cooking. I just grabbed a burger instead. Yum. Grateful indeed!" That's no good. Just say stuff for which you are grateful and what other people would appreciate. (By the way, I work from home, so no traffic for me, and my wife is an excellent cook. I just wanted to clarify that).

Dr. John Sarno

My absolute and most significant breakthrough was reading Dr. John Sarno's *Healing Back Pain.*

Wait, what?

Back pain?

"What in theee hell are you talking about, boy?"

I know what you're thinking. But listen up because this might be the most essential section you will read in this entire book. Seriously.

Let's get started.

Dr. Sarno's book about back pain brought me up to 97% cured. As the name implies, the book is about healing back pain. Dr. Sarno heals debilitating back pain in the most unconventional way.

Instead of back braces, chiro procedures, pills, injections, or surgeries, his method is to lecture you about your back pain.

Huh?

That's right. He lectures about your back pain, and then you're cured.

"Listen, boy. I don't want to be lectured. You better start making sense!"

Before I get into the details, you're probably asking, "How does this relate to heart palpitations?" It does. Just hear me out for a second.

Most people who have severe back pain also have pain all over their bodies. Unfortunately, there are no elbow specialists, no books on pinky pain, and no programs for shoulder pain. All the pain these people have is all the same. It all comes from the same source. That source is your head. Seriously.

Dr. Sarno says that the actual pain is caused by a lack of oxygen to the offending area—whether it's your back, elbow, hands, feet, abdomen, chest, etc. This lack of oxygen comes from—get ready—your suppressed rage. That's right. Your suppressed rage/anger causes this pain.

But you don't have suppressed anger.

No one does.

But you do. You just don't know it.

So, how does this relate to your heart? I don't have any scientific proof other than what Dr. Sarno talks about in his book, *Healing Back Pain*. The book is mostly about back pain and other body pain, such as sciatica. However, he does briefly mention heart palpitations.

My discovery

Although Dr. Sarno doesn't talk much about heart palpitations in his book, I made my discovery quite by accident. The reason I bought his book is because I was having back pain and pain all over my body, including my chest.

I had been successful at reducing my heart palpitations. At the point of reading his book, I barely had any heart palpitations. So, what happened? I had managed to suppress all my symptoms by using pills and breathing exercises. I never really addressed the real problem—my suppressed rage.

When my symptoms of the heart got suppressed by my remedies, I got new symptoms. Those new symptoms were sharp pains all over my body. Not surprisingly, most of the severe pain was in my chest area. When it came across my chest and near my heart, I freaked out. I thought I was having a heart attack.

In Dr. Sarno's book, he calls this affliction TMS. This has had different definitions over time. First, it stood for Tension Myositis Syndrome. Later his definition of TMS was Tension Myoneural Syndrome, and finally, some people called it The Mindbody Syndrome.

Sarno says that for you not to feel the suppressed emotional pain, your body produces physical pain (by way of decreased oxygen) to distract you from your inner rage. Does that make sense? You have emotional pain, but your body doesn't want to recognize it, so it produces actual physical pain. For people like us, it makes our hearts go crazy. We have heart palpitations.

I won't rehash what his book says, but I want you to know that what he says about TMS and back pain also applies to people with heart palpitations. He's written other books that I believe address this very thing. I just haven't read them. All I know is that the information in *Healing Back Pain* brought my condition to a 97% cure. It was quite enlightening.

I realized that maybe I could have some deeply suppressed anger. The beautiful thing is that you don't have to know what that anger is. You just need to know that you have that anger, and that's what is causing your pain. Whenever I had pain in my chest or even heart palpitations, I would say, "That's my TMS acting up." Slowly, my heart palpitations would go away. I finally made the connection between my mind and my heart. It was indeed an incredible revelation for me.

I was on a new path to healing. I had finally found a tool that helped me find a real cure for my heart palpitations. It wasn't just some temporary fix or some way to suppress my symptoms. I finally recognized the emotional pain in my body. Once I realized the emotional pain in my body, my body no longer reacted. I just had to give it recognition.

There is a lot that needs to be discussed on this issue. That's why Dr. John Sarno wrote a whole book on this. I just wanted to let you know that his book was a real turning point for me. I highly recommend you read *Healing Back Pain* or any one of his other books about the mind-body connection. This has worked for me. I kid you not.

I don't have pain anymore and don't have heart palpitations anymore. And if I do, I tell myself that my TMS is acting up, and it goes away.

Hypnosis writing

During my spiritual journey, I decided to see how writing would help with my heart palpitations. I started to do what I call hypnosis writing. Since I've had the condition for over three years, it was ingrained in my head that I had a severe problem. I wanted to reverse that. I wanted to write something that would get into my head that would let me know that I was okay.

This is what I wrote:

"I have a strong and healthy heart."

I repeated that over and over. I filled up a whole notebook page with that. Usually, I would either write a full page or write for five minutes.

This started to make me feel better. It really did. I would write this while listening to music. The idea is to get this mantra into your subconscious, so listening to music while writing seems natural. Besides, listening to music made it seem fun—not a chore.

Later, I embellished my statement to be more specific, so my subconscious brain knew exactly what I was talking about.

This is the second version:

"I have a strong and healthy heart with a normal rhythm."

That sounds more specific to my condition, doesn't it? I could have said "sinus rhythm," but that sounds too scientific. My brain would say, "What the hell are you talking about? Sinus rhythm?" Sometimes it's just better to be unscientific.

I was careful not to make a statement like:

"My heart is as strong as a lion."

I don't know if lions have strong hearts. They may have weak hearts, and they may die of heart attacks all day long. I don't know, so I was careful not to make any comparisons like that. The same goes for athletes.

I almost wrote:

"I have the heart of an athlete."

Again, do athletes have healthy hearts? I don't know. I know they kick off early once in a while. I wanted my statement to be safe and true to me.

So, now I have my new and more specific statement that is safe and pertains to my particular problem.

Every morning, I would set my timer for five minutes and write: "I have a strong and healthy heart with a normal rhythm."

After a while, I started chanting this on my walks in the woods. Whenever I felt a flutter, I would chant, "I have a strong and healthy heart with a normal rhythm." I would chant this about twenty times.

After doing this for a week or two, guess what happened?

I felt great. Things were turning around for me. I felt so great that I modified my written hypnosis.

So, my final chant or written hypnosis is:

"I have a strong and healthy heart with a normal rhythm, and I feel great."

This solidifies the whole thing for me. It's specific and shows my appreciation. This helped me on my walks in the woods. Whenever I climbed up a hill and felt my heart flutter, I would chant, "I have a strong and healthy heart with a normal rhythm, and I feel great."

I just repeated that over and over. Try it and see if it works for you!

Summary

I have come to realize that my heart palpitations were more of a mental problem than a physical one. Even though my symptoms were genuine, the source of those symptoms came from my mind.

However, I do recognize that I was probably deficient in vitamins and minerals like vitamin D and magnesium. And I also acknowledge that I was unhealthy, so removing triggers, eating right, and keeping my body in shape certainly helped with my heart palpitation.

However, the most significant breakthrough for me was that it's all mental. I had many underlying issues. I didn't know I had them. And I still don't know I have them. The breakthrough for me was knowing that my physical symptoms, the heart palpitations, were caused by suppressed emotions such as rage and deep anger.

This is what I learned from reading Dr. Sarno's book *Healing Back Pain*. In his book, he says you only need to be aware of the problem to be healed. And that's what I did with my heart palpitations. I told my mind and body that I was aware that I had suppressed rage. That's all it took — just recognizing it. That's how it works.

And of course, I practiced some other mindful techniques as well, such as meditation, spirituality, gratitude journaling, appreciation of nature, and hypnosis writing.

I firmly believe had I not done any of these mental and mindful practices; I would only be halfway cured. I would still be relying on supplements and questioning whether they were working for me or not. I would always be in doubt

Key takeaways:

- It's all mental
- Meditation helps calm the mind
- Being spiritual allows you to see outside yourself (and your problems)
- Walking in the woods can be peaceful and relaxing
- Having gratitude each day will put you in a calm and confident state of being
- Recognizing that your heart palpitations are caused by suppressed emotions is a critical step on the path to healing
- Talk yourself to being better through hypnosis writing

-7-

If I had to do it all over again.

Knowing what I know now, I would do some things differently. Some things work better than others. While I only included the things that actually worked for me, I'm sure you would like to do something a little easier.

Like I said in the last chapter, as far as I'm concerned, these heart palpitations are a symptom of a mental problem. With that said, my approach would be to attack this problem as if it were a psychological problem. However, that doesn't mean I wouldn't take any supplements or do any other physical exercises.

[At this point, if you're still reading and are interested in the mind-body connection and solution to your heart palpitations, I would suggest you read my second book called: *Conquer Your Heart Palpitations!: Discover the Unconventional Solution for Everlasting Relief.* This book goes much deeper into fixing your head for everlasting relief.]

First, I would get a regular checkup and blood work done just to make sure there isn't some real physical problem—like a loose valve or something. (At the time of this writing, Mick Jagger of the Rolling Stones just underwent surgery to have his heart valve fixed, although he had no prior symptoms). So, it's a good idea to get things checked out at the doctor's office. Just don't get talked into any senseless medication.

I would want to get my magnesium and B vitamins levels checked out. Magnesium is a hard thing to test, but it is possible. I don't know the exact details, but if you read anything by Dr. Carolyn Dean, she will tell you what tests work and what tests don't.

I would also want to get any other levels checked that have to do with the heart. However, I would ignore cholesterol and stuff like that. Doctors love to give you drugs for that, and the jury is still out on that one. There are several books with "cholesterol" and "hoax" in their titles that will make you think twice.

Anyway, I would want to have my potassium and calcium checked, as well. I don't want my calcium too high or potassium too low.

Also, I would have a coronary calcium scan done just to rule out any nasty stuff. I still haven't done this, so that's all I'm going to say about that. The bottom line, I would want to rule out anything physical. When my doctor tells me that "It's all in your head," this time, I will believe her and say, "Okay."

Read books and articles

Once I have been checked out and cleared, I would start reading everything I could about the mind-body connection and maybe some stuff about anxiety. Like I said at the beginning of this book, I don't feel that I have a classic case of anxiety. I don't have the impending doom feeling that everyone talks about. I don't feel like I must escape or that the room is closing in on me. However, I would still read a few books about anxiety just to see what they have to say.

Of course, I would read all of Dr. John Sarno's book, including *Healing Back Pain*. I would totally immerse myself in the concept of TMS. (Today, it is known as The Mindbody Syndrome.) Another good book to read is *The Great Pain Deception* by Steven Ray Ozanich. It's a long read, but he pretty much nails it.

Stop being angry

Knowing what I know now, being upset about my condition only prolongs it. I would stop immediately being offended by anything and everything that would seem offensive. If my heart palpitations happen, I would just let it go and continue working on my program.

Unfortunately, I hear too many people in online forums and on Facebook complain about their condition. I tell them that complaining will only prevent them from getting better. They don't want to hear that. They just want to complain and get sympathy from the other group members.

Don't complain to anyone about your condition. It will only make it worse. They won't understand you, and this will further make you angry. You will suppress this anger, which will, in turn, make you have more heart palpitations. It's a vicious cycle.

Discovering this was a real revelation for me. While I never publicly complained online, I did talk to my wife frequently about it. Her reply was often, "Well, I guess it's something you will have to live with for the rest of your life."

Do you think this made me angry? Shit, yeah! Did I tell her that it did? Hell, no! So, what happened? I just suppressed my anger further and further. Talking about my heart palpitations didn't help.

However, just like Dr. John Sarno mentions in his book, you can go to a therapist to talk about your anger or whatever is bothering you. A therapist is a professional, and you are talking about the cause, not the symptom. The cause is pent-up anger. The symptoms are the heart palpitations. You can talk about what's making you angry, but don't talk about or complain about your heart palpitations (your symptoms).

Therefore, talking to my wife didn't work. Even if she did have a sympathetic ear, I was only talking about the symptoms (my heart palpitations). I wasn't addressing my underlining issues. Only a professional can and should explore those.

Stop watching the news

Often times what's making us angry is not just family and work, but also what's going on in the world. Who dictates our feelings about what's going on in the world? The news. I think the news is the devil incarnate.

The newscasters are demons in disguise. All they do is broadcast hatred and fear. Have you ever noticed that they don't even report the news anymore? It's only their commentary. Their reporting is about thirty seconds long, but their hate-filled blathering goes on for nearly an hour. It's disgusting.

I was two years into my severe heart palpitations before I decided to stop watching the news altogether. I wish I had done it years earlier. The only thing the news did for me was make me fear and hate other people. I woke up one day asking myself, "Why do I hate these people? Where did that come from? Where did that hate and fear come from?" The answer was obvious.

I knew it wasn't from my family. Rarely was it from my friends. I barely heard it at work. The only conclusion was from the news. If someone else was talking about who to hate and fear, where did they get it from? The news.

The news is destructive to the human psyche. Ever since I stopped watching the news, I have felt so much better. However, the destructive nature of the news is long-lasting. I had consumed news regularly for nearly thirty years. That's a lot of garbage to clear out. It wasn't going to happen overnight.

The news made me fear airplanes, traffic, nighttime, liberals, conservatives, the ozone, Mars, the ocean, foreign countries, foreigners, and just about everything else I should have enjoyed as a human being on this planet. But no, I had to be a fool and listen to all the vile that spewed out from the talking heads on the television.

It's not their fault. It's my fault. I listened to them. They can say whatever they want. I just don't have to listen to them, and I won't anymore.

So far, this has been one of the best things I've done in my life. Seriously. I've been consumed by the news. It's awful. I'm sure you've watched your share of the news. It's time to let it go. Believe me; you won't miss a thing.

Stop watching commercial TV

The news isn't the only thing that will rot your brain. Regular commercial television will rot your brain as well. Anything on CBS, NBC, ABC, FOX, UPN, etc., etc. I can't keep track of all the stations anymore. I'm glad I gave this up years ago.

Still, I can't believe how many years of my life I wasted watching this crap. It wasn't until I was in my mid-forties that I finally cut the cord. I wish I had done it a whole lot sooner. I can't believe I used to watch mind-numbing sitcoms with that stupid-ass John Goodman. Ugh! I just want to puke all over my keyboard right now. (Wow, this book has really turned a corner. Hasn't it? Oh, boy.)

Thank goodness for Netflix, Amazon Prime, and a bunch of other streaming channels. I don't have to be relegated to watching stupid sitcoms, nighttime dramas, and fake news shows like 20/20 and Dateline. Are they even around anymore? I don't know. I'm really showing my ignorance (and age) here.

If you want to be in a better mood and heighten your vibration, cut the cord and say goodbye to network/commercial television. Nothing but garbage.

The worst part is that you must sit through those mind-numbing commercials about soda, tile cleaner, and tampons. Ugh! Enough with the tampons! I don't want to know! Ugh! I can't get it out of my head.

And the really worst part is those goddamn fearmongering commercials about some fictitious ailment in which you are supposed to "ask your doctor" about so she can give you some drug in which the side effects mean certain death—in "most cases."

Just turn off the commercial television and live, damn you. Live! (Yeah, this book has definitely gone off the rails. Well, what are you gonna do? Did I tell you that some profits will go to charity? Just remember that.) Commercial television will rot your brain.

Recently, I was watching a free movie on Roku—a free streaming channel, which means there are advertiser supported—which means I'm subjected to mind-numbing commercials. It had been nearly a dozen years since I was willing to watch commercials.

While watching this free movie on Roku, the first two commercials I saw were for "I Can't Believe It's Not Butter" and for Pediasure for children. All poison. I can't believe they are allowed to advertise that shit. Both of those will kill before you know it. Seriously. "I Can't Believe It's Not Butter" is a trans-fat that is (or was) banned in New York. And Pediasure is just pure shit. They'll have to ban that sooner or later. That's the kind of crap you get from commercial television.

Anyway, I gotta move on. We have lots to cover here. Just to bring this whole rant into context: Watching stupid sitcoms where they belittle each other only makes you feel self-conscious, which adds to your anxiety (whether you know you have it or not).

Watching nighttime dramas like hospital/trauma shows only makes you anxious about your own mortality. Stupid shows like 20/20 and Dateline only heighten your anxiety because maybe "this could happen to you." And all the other shows only make you more anxious. This leads to more heart palpitations. Stop watching commercial television! Enjoy a calm movie on Netflix with no commercials.

Limit social media

You may or may not have heard about all the pitfalls of social media. I'm mainly talking about Facebook and Instagram.

These are the places where you get to see everyone's highlight reel and think that what they are presenting is their real life. It's not.

However, you begin to believe that your life sucks. Don't worry; everyone feels that way. That's the way Facebook was designed. Feeling like your life sucks and all your friends are having the times of their lives only heightens your anxiety, inner turmoil, and suppressed anger and rage. This is what leads to your heart palpitations.

Not only that, but now social media is a gateway for all the crap that you are trying to get away from on commercial television. Murders, rapes, incest, wheelchair puppies, protests, politics, etc.

Yes, I did mean to say wheelchair puppies. I've seen way too many puppies on wheels. It's distressing to me. My heart goes out to those paralyzed puppies who must use wheels to get around, but it's just too much for me to bear. Therefore, I must limit my Facebook activity. Just too many wheelchair puppies. So sad. So very sad.

Get away from this shit and feel a whole lot better. I only get on Facebook once in a while but usually stay away.

Limit YouTube videos

I love YouTube because you can find anything on YouTube. This is obviously a blessing and a curse. According to the many videos on YouTube, I'm apparently doing the following all the wrong way:

- Tying my shoes
- Walking
- Breathing
- Drinking water
- Eating mangoes
- Eating avocadoes

These are just a few of the videos that I can think of off the top of my head that are telling me that I am doing something the wrong way. There were plenty of other videos showing me that whatever I was doing was completely wrong. How does this make me feel? It makes me feel like I'm doing everything wrong. Does this raise my anxiety level? My angst? My inferiority? Shit, yeah!

YouTube is great but be careful about the well-meaning people who are trying to help you with every aspect of your life. I watched one video of a man telling me that I've been tying my shoes the wrong way all my life. He had a better technique. Somehow, my method wasn't good enough. This made me shrink inside. Another man told me I was walking the wrong way. Who knew? Now, whenever I walk down the street, I wonder if I'm screwing up my posture because I'm "walking the wrong way."

Some of them are well-meaning, but they can go too far. I learned I was breathing the wrong way, so that helped. But then there are a million videos telling me that I'm not drinking enough water. There is an equal number of videos showing me that I'm drinking too much water. What the hell?

And, of course, I've been eating mangoes and avocadoes the wrong way for years. Oh, boy. Look, I'm not saying these videos aren't helpful. They are. I know how to cut an avocado into chunks without taking off the skin. That's good. However, sooner or later, this stuff can make you a bit neurotic. And that's just the simple stuff. I didn't bother to mention the heavy things like taxes, leaky roofs, pesticides, and a bunch of other stuff.

This should go without saying but stay away from all the negative videos that include politics, "fail" videos, accident videos, celebrity bashing videos, etc. No matter what side of the political spectrum you're on, it's probably a good idea to stay away from anything that involves President Donald Trump. It will only make you more agitated.

Watch fish

To stay calm, I started to watch fish in virtual aquariums. The fish were in actual aquariums; I was just watching videos on YouTube of fish in aquariums. This had a very calming effect on me. Instead of watching "fail" videos, car wrecks, and stupid politicians, I just watched fish videos. Most of them were quite dull, so I only watched them for 20 minutes or so. There were a few coral reef documentaries that were longer and quite soothing.

YouTube has many great aquarium videos. The best thing to do is to sit in a chair for twenty minutes and just watch the fish swim. Just watch them swim. They don't mind. This can be very relaxing.

Stop talking to friends about...

Just like social media, friends can be a great source of anxiety for you. People often commiserate about negative things. Have you ever heard of the term "Misery loves company"? Well, you will find your friends often indulge in negative talk, gossip, and other upsetting things.

Do you know what this does to your psyche? It raises your anxiety, angst, and feelings of being inferior. What does this do? It heightens your sensitivity and causes heart palpitations.

Whenever my friends start going down that road of negative talk, I change the subject or tell them I must get going. I don't have time for celebrity trashing, politics, hating, friend bullying, etc. Let them do it on their own time. I need to be mellow.

Recently, a friend of mine was rattling off every negative news story that came to mind. My response to every one of them was, "That's why I don't watch the news." This dumbfounded him, but it got him to shut up fast.

If you want to have a calm heart—one that doesn't flutter, palpitate, and go erratic—then you need to have a quiet mind and a relaxed soul. Those who thwart your efforts should just be left behind. Your well-being is much more critical.

Stop watching violent and upsetting shows and movies

It seems today that many "TV" programs are getting more graphic. I put TV in quotes because many of these programs are shown on Netflix, but they resemble a TV series that you would see on regular commercial television.

I mentioned earlier in the book how my heart went into an SVT episode when I was watching a show about medieval England. They showed a man being disemboweled with his gut flying out. I had never seen this portrayed so realistically like this before. I know it was fiction, but for some reason, my heart didn't think so.

Another series I started to watch on Netflix and then stopped was *Roman Empire*. Whenever they had sword fights, it was too graphic. For some, this may be high entertainment, but I thought it was just too realistic. I'm more into the movies they made in the 1950s. Even if they had sword fights, they didn't show splattering blood—in slow motion, no less.

Everyone has their own level of what they can handle, so I'm not passing judgment on anyone or even the programs. They can show whatever they want if they have an audience for it, great. But for those of you who suffer from heart palpitations, you should think long and hard about what you consume daily.

It may not be immediate and as visceral as some of my experiences, but it does have an effect. In fact, there was a time I could watch violent television shows, and they had no impact on me. However, the reality is that they did have an effect. It was just slow. It was slowly having an effect. I just didn't know it because I didn't feel anything at the time.

Ever since I cut out violent television programs and movies, I feel much calmer and relaxed. This is so important to finding a cure for your heart palpitations. Remember, your issue built up over time. This isn't something that happened overnight, although it may seem like that.

For me, it seemed very sudden because I had noticed daily heart palpitations immediately after I had my viral infection. I just assumed it was something physical.

I assumed it was only physical because I lost a lot of vitamins and minerals during my antibiotic treatment. I thought the antibiotics screwed up my microbiome. This is all true. But I assumed I could cure heart palpitations just by replenishing my body with vitamins, minerals, and probiotics.

These helped a lot, but there was something more to it. It wasn't until I discovered the mind-body connection from Dr. Sarno. After taking vitamins and other supplements for years, it was clear to me that wasn't the only remedy I needed to explore.

I could write a whole book with studies and statistics, but I won't. I will just say that if you indulge in violent television programs and movies, you should think long and hard about what that is doing to your psyche.

Remember, we have two minds (maybe more). We have our conscious mind and our subconscious mind. Our subconscious sees these violent images as real. That's why your heart will race when you see someone in danger on TV. You, your conscious mind, know it is just a television program. You know that person on screen isn't really in danger. You know that person will be on another episode or another program in the future.

But your subconscious thinks that it is real. That's why you get a physical reaction. You may not notice it that much, but your body does react physically. It does so because your subconscious commands it so. Your conscious mind doesn't have control over your sweat glands or your heart. Your subconscious mind does.

Have you ever woken up from a bad dream with a pounding heart? It wasn't real. You weren't really being chased by a scary monster, but your subconscious thought you were. You weren't really running. You were in bed, lying motionless and asleep. Yet, you woke up as if you had just run a marathon. This kind of scenario has happened to me many times.

Political shows

I like a good political debate, just like anybody else. Whenever there is a video about a hot topic, I am tempted to watch it. Before my moratorium on upsetting programming, I would just watch these hotly debated shows. Today, I am tempted to watch these programs, but I must try very hard to resist. Sometimes I don't succeed. I end up watching some shows about illegal immigrants or college tuitions, etc. When I resist, I feel good about that decision.

These programs are like drugs. Initially, it feels good to watch these shows. But over the long run, you become damaged. And that damage manifests in our bodies in different ways. Some people go into a deep depression, while others get physical pain or heart palpitations.

See a therapist

This is something I hadn't done during my recovery, but I think it would have helped me a lot. If I had to go through this all over again, I would see a therapist.

Whenever I talked to people about my condition, they just looked at me with a blank stare. They didn't know what to say. They were often sympathetic, but they really didn't know what to say. They didn't understand.

However, a therapist would have an understanding ear. They are paid to understand. I wouldn't be looking for sympathy, just understanding. A therapist could help me cope with what was going on in my life and analyze it.

I didn't know there were things in my life I was stressing out about. Of course, I don't want someone to tell me to be fearful of or aware of something I was happy not to know. Sometimes, living in blissful ignorance is ideal. However, as Dr. Sarno pointed in his book *Healing Back Pain*, the anger and rage that we feel are not apparent to us. We are often unaware of this suppressed anger.

Dr. Sarno suggested for severe cases of TMS; one should see a therapist if they can't get past the TMS treatment plan. I would go to a therapist for just a few visits just to talk about the issues that have been building up for many, many years. I'm not someone who consciously dwells on things for too long, so I wouldn't make it a long commitment. I would see a therapist for about six months.

One thing to note about what Dr. Sarno said about TMS is that the people who are the most susceptible are the people who are often kind and caring individuals. Friends and family tell me that I am a good listener. I usually don't do the talking. I just listen. I absorb what people say to me. If they say something I disagree with, I often don't say anything. I'm not one who likes to get into an argument. Unfortunately, this is the type of personality that is susceptible to TMS. (TMS is now referred to as The Mindbody Syndrome).

This didn't really become apparent to me until I started exploring spirituality and "letting things go." While letting things go was good for my well-being and being relaxed, it managed to suppress my anger and rage further. The supplements and physical exercises worked wonders for suppressing my heart palpitations. However, my TMS started to manifest into pain all over my body.

When the pain was in my chest, it just freaked me out because that is where all the vital organs are. I had an equal amount of pain in my legs, feet, arms, shoulders, and neck. That pain was inconvenient, irritating, and excruciating, but I didn't think I was going to die right then and there.

That's the biggest problem with heart palpitations. You think you are going to die. You know your heart is a vital organ. If you had a muscle spasm in some other part of your body, then you just feel inconvenienced. You wouldn't think you were on death's bed. Deep down, you know this. This is why I would see a therapist to help me talk this out.

As you can see, my spiritual journey managed to suppress my anger further. I was letting things go on the outside, but on the inside, I was still angry. This is where recognizing my anger is therapeutic. This is part of Dr. Sarno's therapy.

Get spiritual

I didn't tap into getting spiritual until the later parts of my condition. By this point, I was about 78% cured. However, if I had to do things over again, I would look more into spirituality. Getting spiritual means knowing yourself. It's not about some new religion or something outside of you.

People have a misunderstanding of being spiritual. Being spiritual is not like any mainstream religion. Getting spiritual means having a deeper connection with yourself, your world, and the people in that world. That's it.

Once I realized this, I didn't fear my heart palpitations. I realized that this was just another stage in my journey to wherever I was going. Although I fear the pain and discomfort of death, I don't worry about what comes next. I just feel it is another step in my cosmic journey. Spiritual teachers talk about the human form as being just that—a form taken up by the spiritual being.

Getting spiritual allowed me to appreciate the world around me. I started going on hikes and walks in the woods. I began to enjoy these walks—especially alone, without any gadgets. Whenever I walked with other people or with a music player, I always felt like I missed something.

Stop being a hypochondriac

Information can be useful and evil. Learning more about your health can actually save your life. On the other hand, learning about your health can make you fearful of everything. If you watch enough videos on YouTube, you might never leave your home and look at everything you eat with a tiny microscope.

Since every doctor had made me blatantly aware of my high blood pressure—which averaged around 147/83—I was fearful of everything I put in my mouth. Since there is still a war being waged between vegans and Paleo dieters, I didn't know what to eat. Bread is bad. Eggs are bad. Pasta is bad. Chicken is bad. Everything was bad. I was starting to become a hypochondriac.

Every little pain in my body meant something to me. My calves hurt; I have deep vein thrombosis. My stomach hurt; I have some kind of stomach cancer. My feet hurt; I have incurable gout. On and on it went. I was fearful of everything. What did this do for me?

This made my heart palpitations a whole lot worse.

I wasn't the type of person who went to the doctor for every little thing. In fact, I hated going to the doctor because they always make your condition worse. Doctors did more to raise my blood pressure than anything else. I wasn't one of those hypochondriacs who is always seeking attention. I hated attention and hated seeing the doctor.

However, I read so much about health that I was starting to freak myself out. Was I supposed to get sun? Or not? Should I wear sunscreen or not? Should I eat these shrimps or not? If you watched YouTube, you would see absolute extremes. Many doctors on YouTube will tell not to eat a long list of vegetables for one reason or another. Tomatoes are bad because they are a nightshade vegetable—whatever that means.

Don't take supplements. Take supplements. Vitamin C is bad. Too much vitamin D is bad. Take this kind. Don't take that kind. On and on. Fuck me. What the hell am I supposed to do?

This is where spirituality really helped. It helped me say, "Fuck it, I don't really care about what happens to me. I just want to be peaceful and happy at this moment."

Just like I stopped watching violent shows and heated political debates on YouTube, I also stopped watching "health" shows where some guru was telling me what to eat and what not to eat. I used to follow Dr. John McDougall on YouTube. He has a lot of great information about health and healthy eating.

However, it just got to the point where I didn't know what to do. And his information conflicted a lot with Dr. Eric Berg. I believed in what they both were saying. However, one was vegan, and the other was Ketogenic.

This was a constant conflict. Right now, I am mostly plant-based, with some meat thrown in for good measure. But for a while, I was thinking maybe I was eating too much meat or perhaps not enough. It was all so confusing.

Anyway, I recognized I was a bit of a hypochondriac, thinking every little pain meant something significant. I'm grateful that I found Dr. Sarno's' book about back pain. I plan on reading more books about the mind-body connection. I'd rather read more books about the mind-body connection rather than a book that demonizes a food group, a lifestyle choice, the evils of doctors, or our incredibly toxic environment. If I can control my mind, I feel like I can manage my health.

Summary

There is the easy way, and there is the hard way. The easy way is how you or someone else has done it before. The hard way is how you have no foresight. This chapter is designed to give you some foresight. I focus mostly on mental conditions because that is where I believe this condition lies. It may seem physical—because it is—but you must get beyond trying to "treat" your condition with the physical.

Magnesium and other essential vitamins and minerals are helpful, but I believe they will only get you so far. You are only dealing with the symptoms of the symptom. I didn't say disease because I believe heart palpitations are a symptom of a bigger problem, not a disease in itself that should be treated with medication or other physical modalities.

If I had to do this all over again, I would simply work extremely hard on getting my mind right. I would block out all the negativity in my life. It is actually quite easy to do if you just give it a little effort. We indulge in negativity when we really don't need to. Yes, there will be unfortunate things that go on in your life. But no one is pointing a gun to your head and forcing you to watch television or YouTube and bathe in all that negativity.

No one is forcing you to gossip about people at work or rant about politicians and celebrities on Facebook. You do have a choice. You can decide not to watch violence on TV. You can choose not to watch the local news. It hasn't done anything for you anyway. You can decide to get your head straight. The choice is yours. And your heart is telling you to make that choice.

Takeaways:

- Read books about the mind-body connection
- Stop being angry about yourself, your situation, the world, etc.
- Stop watching the news. Period.
- Stop watching commercial TV. This includes sitcoms, news magazine shows, nighttime dramas.

- Limit social media. Remember, you are only seeing someone's highlight reel. It's NOT their real life.
- Limit YouTube videos—especially ones that are telling you are doing something wrong such as tying your shoes, eating, breathing, drinking water, etc.
- Watch fish in a virtual aquarium on YouTube and relax for twenty minutes a day
- Stop talking to friends about politics, office gossip, your misery, your heart palps, etc.
- Stop watching violent TV and movies. Keep it fun and lighthearted.
- See a therapist. A therapist is a professional who is paid and trained to listen to your problems. No one else is. Not even the people on forums or Facebook.
- Get spiritual. Spirituality means having a better understanding of how you fit in the world. It's NOT a religion.
- Stop being a hypochondriac. Not every little pain means something. Often, it means nothing.

-8-

My daily plan

Below is—or was—my daily plan. Based on the last chapter, this is my hypothetical daily plan. I had done some version of this during my four-year healing process. However, this is an optimized version of it. Since I rarely have heart palpitations or none today, I don't do this exact plan.

So, why do I have a plan like this in here? Well, many people who read a book like this want a specific course of action. So, if I were to recommend a course of action, this would be my recommendation. It's not what I do today, but if I was where I was four years ago, then this is what I would do today.

- ✓ Wake up
- ✓ Drink 20 ounces of water
- ✓ Exercise
- ✓ Take a cold shower
- ✓ Take supplements
    - ○ 200mg of Magnesium
    - ○ 200mg L-Theanine
    - ○ 565mg of Hawthorn Berry

- ✓ Breathing Exercises
- ✓ Write out hypnosis
- ✓ Go for a hike—say chant hypnosis
- ✓ Meditate 25 minutes every morning
- ✓ Avoid all negativity/no complaining
- ✓ Write in Gratitude Journal
- ✓ Eat vegan-centric meals. 1 meat, okay.

This is exactly how it looks. Much of this was written from actual morning procedures I had (and have) in place.

5:00	Wake up
5:01	Remove tape from my mouth (Duh!)
5:05	Drink 16 ounces of water
5:20	Be at the gym working out (light exercise/treadmill)
6:15	Cold shower
6:35	Breathing exercises (5 minutes)
6:45	Read for 15 minutes
7:00	Meditate for 25 minutes
7:25	Write out hypnosis (5 minutes)
7:30	Write in a gratitude journal (2 minutes)
8:30	Eat breakfast
9:00	Start work
2:00	Take a hike

I fill my evenings with getting stuff done, watching relaxing TV, or reading. This helps me calm down before meditating

Throughout the day, I drink herbal/decaffeinated tea.

Wake up

The first order of business is to wake up. Waking up is good. I made sure I had a goodnight's sleep. As discussed, having a goodnight's sleep is very important.

Remove tape

I still sleep with tape over my mouth. This forces me to breathe through my nose, which is the way we should breathe.

Drink 16 ounces of water

It is essential to be fully hydrated throughout the day. I found that drinking lots of water first thing in the morning gets me off to a good start.

Drinking two full glasses of water can be tough if you're not used to it. Once you start doing it, it will become a habit.

One thing I noticed about myself is if I did not drink enough water throughout the day, I would make it up at around 7:00 pm. From seven to bedtime, I would drink two or three glasses of water. Guess what that does? Makes you wake up in the middle of the night to go to the bathroom.

For a while, I had terrible insomnia. I could get to sleep upon going to bed at 9:30, but once I got up at two or three to pee, I could not fall back to sleep.

It's essential to get your water throughout the day. If you eat a lot of fruits and vegetables throughout the day, you don't have to worry about the water so much.

Gym

For me, working out early in the morning before breakfast is the simplest way to get exercise. There is no thinking involved. I'm on autopilot as I go to the gym. I don't have time for excuses. I don't have any interruptions. I just go there and get it done.

I don't make it a long-protracted event. And since I have my condition, I don't want to work out too rigorously. However, I must say that according to mind-body philosophy, you should work out as you usually do regardless of your heart palpitations.

Cold shower

Another benefit of a cold shower is that it wakes you up. If the gym didn't do it for you, this will.

Sometimes if I don't get a good night's sleep, I still feel groggy even after going to the gym. But after taking a cold shower, I really do feel refreshed.

Breathing exercises

Based on the Buteyko breathing program and what I read in Patrick McKeown's books, I practice a few breathing exercises. I don't do them much anymore, but I did this daily to get me to my cure.

The main exercise I did was what they call breath light breathing. Basically, you take very short and shallow breaths to the point you feel like you need to breathe more. It's very uncomfortable, to be honest with you. You feel like you're drowning. But these exercises much helped me with my heart palpitations.

You can find a video on YouTube with this title: Light Breathing Exercises - by Patrick McKeown.

The basic premise of Buteyko breathing is that we are breathing too much. If you are breathing through your mouth, you are breathing too much. Oxygen circulates better when there is more carbon dioxide in your system, so when you breathe out carbon dioxide, your oxygen doesn't flow as much.

Later, I discovered that doing the breathing exercises before going to the gym helped with my workouts at the gym. I didn't always do this. It was a new habit I had to create.

Read

Before I meditate, I like to read to calm myself down. By this time, I had already worked out at the gym and taken a cold shower. I want to lower my heart rate and breathing. Sitting quietly in a chair and reading helps me get into a calm state before meditating.

In fact, I use the same chair that I use to do my mediating for reading. I try not to move too much between reading and meditating. I like to have one action flow into the other.

What do I read? Certainly not *Pet Semetary* or anything that will get me excited. I usually read books about meditation and spirituality. These books calm me down and get me motivated to meditate for more extended periods.

Meditate

As discussed before, I either use a guided meditation or just do it on my own. Right now, my regiment is to meditate for twenty-five minutes on my own. I insert earplugs into my ears, so any outside noise won't distract me. In the Spring, the birds outside my window can get noisy. And traffic is usually distracting.

At one time, I wore blinders for my eyes. But after only a few sessions, I found them to be too distracting. In fact, the outside light doesn't bother me, and it enhances the meditation experience for me because I think about light coming into my soul. So, if it's cloudy out when I start to meditate and becomes sunny, and my room fills with light, I feel like it's light that is entering my body.

Write out hypnosis

As discussed earlier, I have a chant that I write out to hypnotize myself. I won't say much about this here since I've already discussed this. However, doing this has been very beneficial to my recovery.

As mentioned before, I wrote this out for five minutes: "I have a strong and healthy heart with a normal rhythm, and I feel great."

That's it. I just repeat that for five minutes.

Write in a gratitude journal

This is something I do throughout the day, so the morning session is quite short. I just write out what I'm thankful for. That's it.

Eat breakfast

One thing I didn't talk much about is my eating habits. At one time, I was practicing intermittent fasting. This is where you fast for like 20 hours a day. It all depends on who you talk to. I tried it for a few months but didn't see any benefits. My heart seemed the same, and I didn't lose any weight.

The one benefit I did get out of the practice is a good eating habit. While I don't fast for 20 hours, I do have a 14-hour window without eating. My last meal starts at 5:30, and my last bite is at 6:00 pm. I don't eat anything until 8:30 the next morning. No snacks, no treats. This has served me well.

I've been able to sleep a little better. I don't feel as hungry when I go to the gym.

When I do eat breakfast, what do I eat? I'm glad you asked.

It changes a lot during the year. Right now, for the past 6 months, I've been having a bowl of oatmeal with blueberries, raspberries, and bananas. Sometimes, I have strawberries. I got on the oatmeal kick when I started a plan to reduce my cholesterol. Needless to say, it didn't work.

However, eating this way is better than when I was eating two eggs in the morning. One of these days, I will go back to onions and broccoli for breakfast.

Another reason for eating oatmeal is that it is fast and easy to make. I usually use Oat Bran, which cooks in a few minutes.

Supplements

If I were to go through all of this from the beginning, I would only focus on three supplements to help with my heart palpitations.

- ✓ 200mg of Magnesium
- ✓ 200mg L-Theanine
- ✓ 565mg of Hawthorn Berry

Magnesium helps calm the heart and is used in so many body chemical reactions. Magnesium is the first remedy for my heart palpitations, and it helped me to get to about a 25% reduction in my heart palpitations. It made me feel like I was working toward a cure. The only problem was I was limited to how much I could take because of back door bathroom issues.

L-Theanine helps with calming my heart. I usually take it at bedtime. Combined with magnesium, L-theanine puts me right to sleep.

Hawthorn Berry is great for reducing heart palpitations. For me, it doesn't have any side effects or any other effects. I don't even know why people use it other than for heart palpitations.

Walking/Hiking

This has become a daily ritual that I have really come to enjoy. When I first started, it seemed like something I had to do to be healthy. My workouts at the gym were becoming less and less. I was no longer lifting heavy weights and wasn't doing a lot of heavy cardio. I was just walking on the treadmill for thirty minutes. It was all I could do. Otherwise, my heart would go haywire, and I would slip into an SVT. That wasn't pleasant.

A spiritual teacher I had been following talked about connecting with nature and taking walks in the woods. This is what I do every day at around 3:00 pm. Fortunately, I can do this working from home.

If I was working at an office, I would still find time to take a walk during lunch, or I would do it when I got home. In fact, during the few office jobs I had in the past, I did take a 15-minute walk during my lunch break. I did this more to work off my lunch rather than for my heart. This was many years before I had heart palpitations.

Avoid all negativity/no complaining

This one is a biggie. Or, as some people say, "Bigly." Either way, it's huge. Getting your mood right will dictate how your body feels and heals.

Since I've avoided as much negativity as possible, I feel better all around. My heart was feeling a lot better when I first started avoiding negativity everywhere. I stopped watching the news. I stopped engaging in political discussions. I stopped writing nasty reviews for products and books that either didn't work or I didn't like. I stopped griping about the state of the world.

There are two types of complaining. The first type is when you can create real change from your complaining. If people are making noise in a movie theater and you are trying to enjoy the movie, complaining to an usher will bring about immediate change.

The second type of complaining won't bring about any or very little change. This type of complaining is clearly seen in discussing politics and the state of the world. Unless you personally have an action plan to deal with climate change or global warming, then you should probably shut up about it.

Getting all worked up is really, really bad for your health. The only thing you can do is vote for the people who see your point of view. After that, your work is done. You can't do anything else, so just forget about it and let the politicians and scientists duke it out.

This second type of complaining often takes place at the office. If you're pissed that Mary gets all the cool projects, don't complain to some lowly sucker at the water cooler. March yourself right into your boss's office, bang your fist on his/her desk and say, "For fuck's sake, I'm tired of Mary getting all the cool projects. I want some cool projects, or I'm walking. Got that? Good!" If you're not prepared to do that, then shut up.

Complaining to people who can't make a difference is useless noise. Not only is it bad for the environment, but it's terrible for you. It is literally affecting your heart. I can't stress this enough. Your complaining and not accomplishing anything from your complaining only adds to your inner turmoil. These suppressed emotions are what fire off your heart palpitations.

It's not easy to stop complaining, so don't expect to change overnight. But over time, you will get used to it, and you won't give it a second thought. I promise you that if you do this, your heart will feel so much better. It really will.

Eat plant-based meals

I have been practicing veganism for the past ten years. There were periods where I ate no animal products. Today, I limit my animal meals to about four a week. This means four meals with an animal on my plate a week. Not four days a week. Mostly I reserve my animal meals for when I go out to dinner with family and friends.

During the week, my meals are almost all plant-based meals. I have lots of salads, potatoes, pasta, beans, rice, and other fruits and vegetables. My breakfast is usually oatmeal with fruit. No sugar.

Since focusing on plant-based foods, I noticed that my heart feels so much better. When I was in my worse heart palpitations, I was on a high meat-centric diet. The years prior, I was vegan for about three years.

My first major attack happened when I ate a double bacon cheeseburger from Wendy's along with a Dr. Pepper and fries. By the way, just so you don't misunderstand me, I'm not saying that Wendy's is one of those top restaurants I referred to earlier. What I'm saying is that I got used to eating meat and stopped my vegan habits.

My real breakthrough in discovering how good eating a plant-based diet was for my heart palpitations was when I stopped eating eggs for breakfast. The effect was immediate. I didn't stop eating eggs because I thought it would help me with my heart palpitations, so no placebo effect there. No, I stopped eating eggs for breakfast because my doctor said my cholesterol was too high and that I should take steps to control it.

I went back to what I knew worked, and that is to eat plant-based foods. When I went vegan, I shed ten pounds in three weeks without even thinking about it. I wasn't one of those tub-of-lards where ten pounds doesn't mean much. After I lost those ten pounds, I was still only six pounds overweight. That was a big deal. It's not easy to lose those last couple of pounds.

Anyway, I stopped eating eggs for breakfast and switched to plant-based foods. I would eat beans, cucumbers, red peppers, bananas, etc. As I said, the effect was immediate. I noticed significantly fewer heart palpitations. Instead of a hundred a day, I had about fifty a day. That was a big deal for me.

However, I never went full-throttle on plant-based eating. There were a lot of factors, but one was all the good restaurants. I liked going out with friends and having fun. Eating plant-based foods in a restaurant is nigh impossible. So now, I just reserve my meat-eating to mostly the weekends. I still have a plant-based breakfast and lunch. It's only when I go to a restaurant that I get a lobster or something.

Summary

That's pretty much what I had been doing and what I would be doing if I started all over. Now, I'm at a place where I don't need to do all the stuff I mentioned. Although I should do those things for overall health, I don't feel an urgency. For instance, I only do my breathing exercise a few times a week. I don't eat vegan all week. I don't take magnesium every day. I don't chant or write my hypnosis chant.

However, I still drink lots of water (it's excellent for weight loss). I still go to the gym every day. I still put tape on my mouth. I still take other supplements that may or may not help with my heart palpitations. I still take hikes. I still meditate. I still take cold showers.

This is the power plan I would do. Other things can be done, such as what I mentioned in this book, but I wanted to show you a simple, doable plan. I mean a feasible plan for me and my lifestyle. Your situation may be different.

In the end, you must figure out what works for you. But I should warn you not to cut corners. Getting over heart palpitations isn't as simple as taking a pill. I wish it was. You must attack your problem from multiple angles.

The most important thing to remember is that you did something or something happened to you to get you to where you are now. It may have built up over time. You can't expect to get rid of your problem overnight by just taking magnesium.

In my case, I know a bunch of stuff built up over time. I wasn't eating well. I had a crappy attitude about life. I had stressors such as moving, no job, renting a crappy home, being overweight, and a bunch of other shit. I had a lot of negativity in my life. I bathed in the nightly news. I watched highly charged political videos on YouTube. I watch "fail" videos, plane crashes, pranksters, dangerous stunts, etc. I was drowning in negativity and despair. No wonder my heart was freaking out.

I had a lot of anxiety, but I just didn't know it. Other than my heart palpitations, I didn't have the classic signs of an anxiety attack. I didn't feel any impending doom or the need to escape where I was. None of that.

In the end, I realized that I needed to fix my head and fix what was going into my head and body.

Key Takeaways:

- Create a daily plan and stick to it

- Eat a healthy breakfast

- Try plant-based eating

- Drink lots of water

- Keep positive thoughts

-9-

Final Words

My experience

I want to say a few final words before we part ways. I want to emphasize that the tips, tricks, and strategies are based only on my experience. There are many ways to attack your problem. You've probably searched for them. That's why you're reading this book.

It never hurts to seek out more and more sources. There is a ton of other stuff I could have put into this book that I researched and read online. However, my goal was only to present my experience, not what I heard from others. That's their experience, not mine.

Focus on a positive image

If there is one thing that I learned in all of this is that having a crappy attitude will get you nowhere. When your heart palps get you down, try to stay positive. When I was at the height of my heart palpitation episodes, I would curse the world. I would bang my fist on my desk, and I would stamp my feet. Guess what? It did me no good. It only hurt my progress.

Once I adopted a positive attitude about this whole thing, I began to see improvement. Not only did I feel better physically, but my new positive attitude opened my eyes to new therapies that I had never considered. I put my full faith in them with a positive attitude. Some worked, and some didn't.

Continue to believe that it's mental, not physical

When I focused on the physical aspect of my problem and attacked it with pills, diet plans, and exercises, I progressed only a little. Those things helped to a certain point, but other strange things began to occur. The more my heart palpitations went away, the more the pains and other discomforts came about.

It wasn't until I discovered that this is a mental problem—just as much as a physical one—that I started to see real progress. When I began to believe these heart palpitations were a symptom of something else and not a disease in itself that I started to see real progress.

These heart palpitations were my body crying out and telling me something was wrong. I was living a lifestyle that wasn't healthy. I was putting toxic food in my body and harmful information in my head. My heart palpitations were the result.

I consider myself lucky that this is how my body chose to express itself. Other people have much worse problems, such as skin problems, cancer, chronic pain, etc. I look at this as a blessing rather than a curse. I used to look at it as a curse, but thanks to my new positive attitude, I see things differently.

I've done a fair amount of research into all things about health. Most of our problems come from within us. These are often called autoimmune diseases. The body attacks itself. I don't consider heart palpitations as an autoimmune disease, but it is our bodies telling us something is wrong.

This problem didn't come from outer space. We didn't catch it on the African continent. And we weren't necessarily born with it (although it's possible).

Speaking of being born with it: when I was very young, I was told by my doctor that I had a heart murmur. This had always been in the back of my mind all through my life. Anytime I felt anything in my heart, I would think back to the days when my doctor told my mother that I had a heart murmur. This really clouded my thinking, and overall, it wasn't right. However, I chose to ignore all that on my road to recovery.

Wonderful time

We live in the most wonderful time in all of history. We have every convenience our ancestors could only dream of. We have everything we ever need at our fingertips. We can have nearly anything we want shipped from Amazon in just a few days. We can listen to almost any song on Spotify. We can watch all sorts of crazy videos on YouTube. And we can watch almost any movie ever made on Netflix and many more streaming services.

But the news and other pundits on TV (e.g., celebrities, talk show hosts, and other know-it-alls) would have you think we live in absolute HELL. The sky is falling. Everything is a disaster, and every little thing "could happen to YOU."

I could go on and on with my rant, but I'm sure you get what I mean. It's time that you realize that we live in a beautiful world. Only you can choose how you live in it. You can choose to indulge in toxic foods and toxic media, or you can choose to do the opposite.

We have so many choices. When I grew up, we only had seven or eight channels for watching TV programs and movies. I watched stupid sitcoms because that's all there was.

I would shoot myself if I were forced to watch one of those sitcoms today. They are so demeaning. And we had to watch the news if we wanted to know what was going on. We didn't have a lot of choices back then.

Today, you can watch anything on YouTube. (Don't make it harmful like "fail" videos, high tension politics, or plane crashes, and other disasters). You have so many choices. Watch videos about cool science experiments, nature shows, success stories, how to improve yourself, and so on. There are no excuses for choosing to indulge in toxic media.

We live in a wonderful world. If you don't believe that, then you really need to stop watching the news. Anyone who has stopped watching the news knows that we live in a wonderful world and in the most wonderful time in history.

When I grew up, you had to spend up to $16 on an album that contained 45 minutes of music on eight to ten songs. Today, for $9.99 (or free), you can listen to Spotify and have nearly every song you can think of. Do you have any idea how much Grateful Dead I've been listing to? It's amazing, and I am so grateful for that. Yes, major pun intended! Be grateful for Spotify.

And my car has SiriusXM Radio, so I can listen to more Grateful Dead on what channel? Guess? The Grateful Dead channel! How great is that? And I don't pay for it. I bought the car used, and SiriusXM had been previously installed and has been still active for the past 5 years. And I am so grateful for that. My car is old, but I don't want a new car.

It's a wonderful world, I tell you. The more you realize that the better your heart will feel. I promise you that.

Don't read too much about health

You should know the basics about good health, but reading and watching too much can make you very anxious, and you may not even realize it. No matter what health kick you're on, there will be someone somewhere telling you all the dangers of what you're doing.

Eating too many bananas? You're gonna die. Enjoy eating back fat? You're gonna die. Not breathing properly? You're gonna die. Not drinking enough water? You're gonna die. Eggs? Forget it. You're gonna die! No matter what you do, you're gonna die. Shower too hot? You're gonna die. Corn? Bacon? Bread? Milk?

Die! Die! Die! Die! Everything is gonna kill us. So, you might as enjoy living; stop thinking about dying.

I know from my experience that knowing too much about what's gonna kill me will kill me faster than what they are telling me what's gonna kill me. In other words, the stress and anxiety about being healthy is making me unhealthy.

Keep doctor's visits to a minimum

Doctors have an excellent way of freaking you out—except when you visit them for heart palpitations. Then they just shrug their shoulders. Do you know why that is? Because there are no profitable drugs to treat heart palpitations.

Doctors will always find some drug to treat whatever you're visiting them for. It's not entirely their fault. As a society, we have come to expect to get a pill every time we visit a doctor. In fact, if we don't get a pill, we complain, cry, stamp our feet, and go visit another doctor.

However, one of the things that doctors do that annoys me is getting on my case about my blood pressure. There is little scientific proof that high blood pressure causes any disease. It's just a symptom of overall bad health. So, giving me a toxic drug to treat a symptom is like resetting the "check engine" light without addressing the real problem.

There are numerous stories where people went in for a benign physical exam (i.e., requested by an employer or school). They were then told of some horrible disease (i.e., cancer or diabetes) when there really wasn't one present. Look it up.

And the whole preventive care is kind of bullshit. Your body will tell you what's wrong with you. It is up to you whether you choose to ignore it. But having some super electron microscope find some "thing" in the far reaches of your body and then get a round of toxic chemicals to treat it doesn't make any sense to me—and a lot of others.

I'm not saying you don't go to a doctor, but I am saying they aren't the friends you think they are.

Anyway, those are my final words. Thank you for reading this book. If you want to reach out to me with any questions and concerns, please email me at AustinWintergreen@gmail.com

May I ask you a small favor?

If you enjoyed reading this book and would like other people to benefit from the information in this book, could you please review my book on Amazon and/or Goodreads.com?

Thank you!

Your review will help other heart palpitation sufferers find solutions to their problems. This is what helped me!

Click here to write a review on Amazon

Click here to write a review on Goodreads

About the Author

Austin Wintergreen is just an ordinary guy. He's 51 years young, and he lives with his wonderful wife and five daughters in Scottsdale, Arizona. When he's not working, he can be found sailing and fishing whenever the mood strikes him. He also loves spending time with his two dogs Chip and Dip. An avid skier, he and his wife take to the mountains of Colorado in the winter. They also split their time between Scottsdale and New York City.

Made in United States
North Haven, CT
17 March 2023

34225349R00107